Deconstructing the Interview

T0177583

Deconstructing the Interview

Duncan Harding PhD MRCPsych

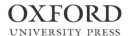
OXFORD
UNIVERSITY PRESS

OXFORD
UNIVERSITY PRESS

Great Clarendon Street, Oxford, OX2 6DP,
United Kingdom

Oxford University Press is a department of the University of Oxford.
It furthers the University's objective of excellence in research, scholarship,
and education by publishing worldwide. Oxford is a registered trade mark of
Oxford University Press in the UK and in certain other countries

First Edition published in 2018

Impression: 1

Published in the United States of America by Oxford University Press
198 Madison Avenue, New York, NY 10016, United States of America

British Library Cataloguing in Publication Data

Data available

Library of Congress Control Number: 2018942722

ISBN 978–0–19–876819–7

Printed in Great Britain by
Ashford Colour Press Ltd, Gosport, Hampshire

Oxford University Press makes no representation, express or implied, that the
drug dosages in this book are correct. Readers must therefore always check
the product information and clinical procedures with the most up-to-date
published product information and data sheets provided by the manufacturers
and the most recent codes of conduct and safety regulations. The authors and
the publishers do not accept responsibility or legal liability for any errors in the
text or for the misuse or misapplication of material in this work. Except where
otherwise stated, drug dosages and recommendations are for the non-pregnant
adult who is not breast-feeding

Links to third party websites are provided by Oxford in good faith and
for information only. Oxford disclaims any responsibility for the materials
contained in any third party website referenced in this work.

Foreword

It is without doubt that Duncan Harding has written here a timely and important book that will be of help to many people. As Dr Harding points out, being interviewed is something that we all have to go through. Managing expectations, anxiety and performance are, therefore, clearly critical to success. Perhaps as important within professional interviews today, which tend towards a more standardized format, is the art of being yourself and using that to your advantage within the interview setting. Having sat on many interview panels, I am all too aware that in addition to competence and a requisite skillset, what the panel is looking for is a real person with whom to engage; with whom one could imagine working; who could make a real and positive contribution to a team. I think Dr Harding's new book should help in enabling the reader to shine through in the interview process, a factor that is critical to success. The task is made all the easier for the reader by the style of personal accompaniment that characterizes Dr Harding's own writing, not something that is easy to deliver and for which he should be warmly commended.

Dr Matthew Patrick
Chief Executive of South London and Maudsley NHS Foundation Trust

Acknowledgements

I would like to thank Dr Chris Chan for her support, thoughts, and reflections. This book is dedicated to my grandfather, Mr Frank Brown, a man who knew the value of hard work, and who found peace within his own authentic life narrative.

Find me at www.deconstructivity.com and @duncanharding

Detailed contents

PART 1

PSYCHOLOGICAL PROCESSES

CHAPTER 1

The road ahead

CONTENTS

Setting the scene

The job interview is an important hurdle and milestone in all of our lives and careers, regardless of background, profession, specialty, or level. It is a psychologically charged event that affects everyone, and as a psychiatrist I felt well placed to tackle this topic from a fresh perspective. *Deconstructing the Interview* is a book aimed primarily at health practitioners, in all levels of training, but is also designed to be useful for *anyone* doing a job interview. This is possible because there are common psychological elements in all interviews—the interview is a highly charged encounter with similar psychological stressors, baggage, and drivers, in all walks of life. Indeed, I believe that the generic strategic approach is what makes this book useful; and that by taking a step back from the intricacies of our specific profession or specialty we can address core issues from a different perspective that might significantly improve our overall interview performance.

The first part of this book will consider those psychological processes and factors that play a part in our interview performance. We will explore our thoughts, motives, and underlying beliefs, and work together to unpick these—thereby developing an access point for unravelling the psychological baggage and barriers that may be holding us back from our full interview potential. We will start to develop a framework of psychological understanding that will help us deal with interview failure, a painful fact of life that we all have to face at some point, and will also enable us to construct a scaffold on which we can start to develop our interview process skills (in Part 3). We will consider stress and anxiety, and develop methods in reframing these into something that can actually be useful in our future interviews. We will bring this all together by considering our confidence and self-belief, and work towards optimizing these and moving towards the best that we can be.

In the second part of this book we will be considering pragmatic approaches to interview preparation and the interview itself, in the context of our new psychological framework of understanding. We will discuss practical issues such as rehearsal strategies, psychological preparation both during rehearsal and before the interview itself, reality checking, and body language. We will think about empathy—our connection with the interviewer, and will consider ways to unpick and optimize this. We will spend time working on our situational awareness, how this can be improved, and how it can add significantly to our overall performance. We will think about our presentation, both in what we wear and how we come across overall, in the context of the psychological drivers and factors at play in both the interviewer and interviewee. We will consolidate all this by reviewing and refining our practices and processes, and find ways to optimize these.

Just as in my previous book in this series, *Deconstructing the OCSE*,[1] here we will not be concerned with the specific content required for a given interview—the content, i.e. the actual answers to interview questions, is assumed knowledge or information that should be sought elsewhere. Here, we are concerned with the processes that underlie our interview performance—these are those non-technical skills that demonstrate confidence, professionalism, non-verbal communication skills, and empathy to the interviewer to name but a few. We will discuss the value of forming an authentic narrative and consider our approach to unknown facets of the interview: the wild cards. In the third and final part of this book we will work together to develop our underlying process skills within the context of our mutually developed psychological framework of understanding. In this final part of the book we will also develop generic skills and strategies that might be useful for any interview hurdles we face.

Clinical interviews

Health practitioners, especially medical staff, attend job interview after interview as they progress onwards through their career. Medical and surgical training has become more streamlined in recent years, so it is more likely that candidates for a given interview will have very similar competencies and attainments in their portfolios—although a few people may stand out, with intercalated PhDs and suchlike, the playing field is much more level than in the past. Therefore, it is critical that candidates perform to their absolute best potential in the more nebulous aspects of the interview—the non-technical process skills. With a strong refined and focussed baseline of process skills, the candidate can be confident that they are as competitive as possible in all aspects of the interview process. Interviews are judged relative to other candidates once you have fulfilled the minimum requirement for appointment, so it is very important to optimize all facets of performance. This book will help you to tune up your interview processes.

Many facets of interview performance naturally improve with more interview practice, especially content and knowledge-based factors relevant for a specific field or specialty. The interviewee starts to learn how to traverse these rocky waters and develops their own style of approach for success. In this book, I will suggest some tips and strategies that may be helpful in the form of generic skills—these can be applied in any interview situation. However, sometimes negative experiences during an interview, or a lack of success, can actually increase stress and anxiety and can lead to a deterioration in subsequent performances—this book will help you kick any negative psychological baggage into touch so that you are not overly burdened by any unsuccessful prior experiences. We will also work on ways to move past negative experiences during the interview itself, so that the negativity and disappointment is reframed and packaged up without colouring your subsequent performance in that interview.

There is a growing trend, in healthcare interviews, for a standardized process that is fair and similar for all—an extreme version of this are some of the current medical and surgical specialty trainee interviews, in which the questions are often pre-published and the interviewers literally stick to the script. In this age of standardized clinical interviews, it is even more important to find an edge in your performance that goes beyond the content itself. Indeed, with pre-published questions every candidate will be walking into the room armed with model answers covering most if not all of the required content—so what will make you stand out? This book will help you to refine and focus your process skills, so that you will present yourself in the best way possible to the interviewers, and thereby maximize your chances of success in competition with your colleagues.

A modular, dynamic skillset

We carry skills into our interview with us, and employ these skills as required. Many of our skills are innate, passive, process skills, learnt and employed over many years and perhaps in several previous interviews. These process skills are absolutely critical and this book will help you to distil and refine these in a mindful, psychological way. Other skills are based in content, perhaps the content required for a given profession or type of interview. These content skills are also critical for interview success and this book will help you to process these skills from context-specific to modular, reforming them into something that could be utilized and employed in a more generalized way. The content skillset should be dynamic, i.e. it should adapt and respond in real-time to a form fit for purpose. This book will help you to transform skills into a more dynamic form.

Anecdotes and exercises

I will use anecdotes and real-life examples throughout the text, from my own experiences and following discussion with colleagues. This will give a 'human face' to the narrative, and will aid your understanding and recall of the concepts within. I will also use exercises throughout, to add a more interactive element to the text, and to improve the learning experience.

A new perspective

Addressing different schools of interview allows us to overtly approach our own interview with a change in perspective, and I believe that change in itself is good in this highly competitive psychological encounter. A change in perspective allows us to approach our obstacle from a different angle—we will not lose any of the naturally evolving content and knowledge-based factors previously attained, but we will be approaching the encounter with a fresh, clean page. The psychological cupboard will be spring-cleaned, and although we will retain all the positive facets previously attained, and thereby not throw the baby out with the bathwater, we will have the cognitive space to reframe negative psychological facets and factors. We will also have a new, clean slate, allowing us the cognitive space to work on our process and non-technical interview skills from a psychological perspective, to refine and optimize these so that we are the best we can be. This book will help you to change your perspective.

Rebooting the system

So, in this book we will take a journey into previously uncharted territory, we will be straying outside of our comfort zones and refining our core interview performance in a new landscape and perspective. We will be mining down into our psychological makeup and extracting the core elements that underpin our non-technical skills, human interactions, and decision-making processes; building a new and robust psychological framework and infrastructure, onto which we can construct a refined process skillset that will improve our core functioning. With this new operating system, powered by a new engine, we can apply our content and knowledge base in a stronger and better way, with the confidence that we are as competitive as possible. We are not trying to drive the same car faster—we are driving a new and faster car.

Reference

1. Harding, D. (2014) *Deconstructing the OCSE*. Oxford University Press, Oxford.

CHAPTER 2

Ground zero

CONTENTS

Starting point

Here we begin the journey into our psychological processes, and we start by considering who we are, what brought us to this point, and why we are here. This is not dissimilar to an opening question in the interview and it is core knowledge that is essential for us, as well as being of interest to the interviewer. Perhaps you know the answers to these questions, and in a way we all do since not knowing these basic things would be terrifying—who we are and why we are here are questions rarely asked, they are assumed knowledge and essential for our peace and wellbeing. At certain times in life, tragedy and adversity in the external world might push us to the point when we are forced to ask ourselves these core questions, when we are forced to question the grounding principles of our core existence. The interview is not such a tragedy, but this is a good time to consider our psychological makeup from the ground up. This is our ground zero, and in this chapter we will begin our processes of psychological dissection and reconstruction.

The good candidate

What makes a good candidate? How do we know that we are a good candidate? Is that important? From the perspective of the interviewer, a good candidate is a person who primarily fulfils the necessary criteria needed to succeed in the job, while also being a person they might get on well with and one who would fit well into the workplace. There may be other less overt factors at play, such as a need to fulfil certain recruitment goals, but given that every job should be a level playing field we won't concern ourselves with that now. Indeed, we won't spend too much time worrying about what the good candidate might look like from the perspective of the interviewer—instead we will consider what makes a good candidate from our own perspective, the interview candidate.

It could be said that the same factors make a candidate 'good', whether from the perspective of interviewer or interviewee, and perhaps from a more objective standpoint that is indeed the case. We need to tick all the boxes, we need to get on well with our colleagues and mould seamlessly into our new environment, but in some ways those things are beyond our control at the point of the interview. They are implied, and we can give the impression that they are all fulfilled, but really the only thing we can hope to do at an interview is perform the very best that we can. A good candidate, from the perspective of the candidate, is simply one that performs as best they possibly can on the day. If we achieve this, then we should be happy.

It is, however, useful to keep in mind what the interviewer would think of as a good candidate, and whilst we should never try to be that person, we can mould ourselves into a shape that fits. We can frame our answers in a way that will be attractive to the interviewer, but we must do so in a way that remains authentic. Therein lies an interesting paradox in interviews. Most interviews will be for a job a person aspires to, beyond their normal comfort zone, a new endeavour; we need to prove that we possess the skills and mettle to be successful in this new role in life, that we will fit in as seamlessly as possible—but to rise to the challenge of a new job we are stepping outside of our comfortable 'authentic' selves and aiming for something higher. In a sense, we are by definition moving into a role that would not fit us like a comfortable slipper, because if it did then perhaps this would not be such an exciting job to aspire towards. This is a balance, and a good candidate will be able to present as authentic whilst recognizing that they are stepping beyond what might be considered comfortably authentic to them. This is a new challenge, a new chapter in our story, and whilst we will retain the qualities that got us to this point in life, we will also recognize our infallibility, we will embrace our humility, and we will work hard to fit into this new role.

A good candidate is an authentic candidate, but what is authenticity? How is authenticity communicated to the interviewer? We will consider this in more detail later (see Chapter 15), but for now consider yourself as a collection of authentic building blocks, rather than authentic as a whole. Consider the facets of your skillset and personality that speak truly to your ethical standpoint and moral code—these are the pieces of you that stack up into the authentic person waiting outside of the interview room. These are the facets of you that need to be disseminated to the interviewer, presented to them within their collection of questions. What are your core values and how do these relate to the specific question being asked? You don't want to be wholly moralistic, but an injection of your authentic building blocks is useful in an interview and will stand you in good stead with the interview panel. Not everything is driven by one's moral standpoint, but perhaps it is a core facet of you that, for example, children should be held at the centre of all decisions around family care, and if so that might be a powerfully authentic opinion to drop into an interview question about family care structures. If you accept that this might be useful, then you already have a piece of preparatory work that would be relevant for any potential job interview—reflecting on your authentic building blocks, perhaps writing them down, and then rehearsing how they might be moulded into an answer that would make sense in this particular job interview.

Being self-aware

Much of this book is about becoming more self-aware, but in a way that takes us outside of our own heads and into the world around us. During an interview, and in the weeks before, we will inevitably exist primarily within the confines of our mind, amongst our abilities and limitations, as we try to prove to the interviewer that we are the right and best person for the job. However, us, as beings in the interview, are more than our collected thoughts and skills—we are sitting in a room, probably anxious and sweating, on an uncomfortable chair being scrutinized by others. We are the collection of all these things, we are our thoughts and internal being as well as the interfaces we make with the outside world, and we need to see ourselves as such. We need to step outside and see ourselves from across the room to truly be self-aware. How do we appear to those around us? How are we filling the space? How are we reacting? What is our body language communicating? We need to see beyond the thoughts we have and the words we say, we need to view our performance as a whole and be aware of all the tiny things the interview panel might notice. We will work hard in this book to try to operate externally, to put ourselves into the interview space and observe all aspects of our presence and performance, and also place ourselves into the mind of the interviewer. But perhaps the best place to start, in terms of self-awareness, is inside, right here. Why do we want this job? How does this fit into our life narrative, our story so far? What would it mean to be successful? Unsuccessful? Is there a Plan B? We must first explore the inside, understand and reflect as best we can, perhaps discuss and debate with a friend, and then move into the external space and be aware of our existence in the interview as a whole.

Authenticity is an essential aspect of being self-aware—being aware of what makes us authentic, and how to bring those authentic building blocks into the interview space in a way that makes sense to the interviewer. We need insight into what the interviewer requires and wants, and with that insight we can mould and present our authentic elements to them. An interview should never be 'playing a game', in the same way a first date shouldn't. If we play a game at the start, and inauthentically present things that we imagine the other person would like to see, then we will always be playing a game. An interview is the start of a new chapter in life, and we need to embark upon this adventure with truth and authenticity.

What is the truth of us as a person? We can perhaps think of our personality as a collection of 'sub-personalities', the building blocks of personality that all join together to make up the whole. We might sit down and think about what those building blocks are. At what stage in our life did they develop and how do we tend to show and employ them in life? On a first date, or in a stressful social situation, we might find ourselves falling back to default of 'humour', and our humorous sub-personality might become dominant. We might find that we tend to define ourselves by a particular aspect of our personality, for example 'the comedian' or perhaps 'the intellectual', and whilst humour might successfully get us through most situations in life, it could be that the interview is not one of those times. We need to work on our sub-personalities, become comfortable with the concept of them forming our whole being, then apply those aspects of our personality as appropriate in the interview.

Indeed, what is an interview? An interview is an interchange of views, it is the formation of a collaborative space with another person to see if your particular view can fit with theirs. In order to do that, we need to have a clear idea about what our views actually are, and how we can package and apply them in this situation. Also, which of those views on life intersect with our core beliefs and authentic selves? It might be that the views of the interviewer, or company as a whole, clash terribly with our own views and values, and in this case perhaps they are unsuccessful in the interview for us rather than vice-versa.

Is an interview just a game that we must play? I would suggest that even if there are aspects of game playing, and even if we might develop rote answers and skills that can satisfy all the potential games an interviewer might set, one aspect of the interview is essential and certainly not a game: are you a person they would like to work with? Are you a nice person, who might be funny but not too funny, who will fit in and be a loyal and respectful colleague? This aspect of the interview is not a game, it is a truthful meeting of individuals in life and common ground needs to be sought out. So ground zero, regardless of the type of interview, is that we need to bring truthful aspects of ourselves into the interview space, and see if they fit with the other side of the table. I suggest that this is a good starting point, and whilst being truthful and authentic in an interview might feel terribly exposing and unsafe, I think that packing aspects of our authentic selves, alongside parts of our personality, are good foundations for building a bedrock of interview skills that will keep us stable and grounded during this stressful psychological meeting of minds.

Core internal state

An interview is designed to push us to our emotional and intellectual limits, to push us out of our comfort zone and see how we respond under pressure. From the perspective of the interviewer, they want the candidate to perform authentically and to be as good as they can be, but they also want to gently push the candidate to their limit. An interview that goes well, from the perspective of the interviewee, should feel emotionally and intellectually challenging, and indeed if we are not feeling challenged then perhaps we are not performing to the best of our abilities. Given this, then it also follows that at moments when we are pushed to the limit our façade drops and our core internal state shines out into the interview space like a beacon. At points of high pressure, the truth of us will blast out into the interview space, sometimes by the things we say but more often by the way we come across. The small non-verbal gestures, the wringing of fingers, the closed defensive body language, our relaxed arrogance—all of these are poker tells, and all must be kept mindfully in check throughout the interview.

That said, it would be better if our core internal state was one that would be appealing to the interviewer, for example, just the right amount of anxiety for a job that would be a step up in life. It might be that our relaxed arrogance is just an internal defence to protect us from the anxiety of a job that might actually be very stressful and challenging, at least at first. Whether we can identify a defence like this or not, I suggest that it is useful for all of us to reflect on how we really feel about this job and new chapter in life, and to try and break down any defences that might have developed in the name of self-preservation. I would say that this is a time in life to exist in the anxiety that this new position potentially brings, at least in the period when we are preparing for the interview, and to allow ourselves the indulgence of feeling unsure and worried about what the future might bring. If we can do this in the days and weeks before the interview and find peace in that, then we are less likely to express our fear and anxiety in the interview itself. Remember, it is important to be *mindfully anxious* about a new chapter in life, indeed such grounded anxiety is probably attractive to the interviewer. In contrast, being arrogantly relaxed or unconsciously anxious is a much less attractive proposition. Let us choose to be mindfully anxious.

We will now dissect into our core internal state by exploring our good and bad qualities, how these relate to this particular job, and how they are potentially related to each other (see Exercise 2.1).

EXERCISE 2.1 **THE GOOD AND THE BAD**

It's not unusual to be asked to list your good and bad qualities in a job interview, and even if that question isn't explicitly asked it's essential to have a good understanding of these in the interview. Being more explicitly aware of our positive and negative attributes will help us find ourselves, but also will furnish us with a useful interview answer should the question arise. In this exercise we will make a list of the good and the bad as they relate to particular facets relevant for this particular interview. By *facets* I mean individual skills or qualities relevant for this job, for example 'leadership', 'team-working' etcetera. Here we will be brutally open and honest, perhaps more so than might be possible or desirable in the interview itself, but open enough to pry into all those defended psychological corners and recesses. Ideally, any bad quality needs to have the ability to be moulded into a positive one, and you can also use this exercise to help with that. Remember though, bringing something 'bad' to an interview should be a bad behaviour that can be modified into good, not something inherently bad about you as a person—so, for example, you have 'boundless enthusiasm so sometimes lack focus' rather than being 'lazy and bored'.

Take a piece of A4 paper and divide it into three columns. Label the first column 'facet', the second 'good', and the third 'bad'. In the first column list some skills or qualities relevant for this job, such as 'leadership' and 'team-working'—list only a few facets in the first column leaving

---

(continued)

room to work on the good and bad for each. Next to the first facet, in the second column write something good about yourself, and in the third something bad. If the facet was 'leadership' you might write 'good people skills and communication' in the second column, and 'uncomfortable telling others what to do' in the third. In this worked example the 'bad' quality can be presented to the panel with mindful awareness—you can tell them that you struggle with telling others what to do, but are working on ways to communicate this as fairly as possible by refining your people skills. The good quality and bad qualities are linked in this way—try to find good and bad qualities, linked to a particular facet, which balance and have the potential to feed into each other. So you can list the good and the bad, but use the good to offset the bad. Draw arrows between the good and bad to indicate how they are linked; perhaps annotate the arrow to indicate, for example, 'improved communication reduces my sense of discomfort'.

For the next facet below, e.g. 'team working', find good and bad things about yourself and consider how these balance and feed into each other. You might find that your good and bad qualities from the facet above also have relevance for this facet, for example, communication skills are essential team working attributes. Find common ground in your good and bad qualities between the different facets, but try to frame them in slightly different ways depending on the particular facet. In this example, leadership and team working employ similar building blocks of skills and qualities, but are distinct entities. When thinking about our good and bad qualities, and indeed when speaking about them in the interview, it is useful to properly dissect into them and present them as such. In that way, you have a good understanding of how your good communication is important for leadership and also for team working, in a slightly different but distinct way. Think about the balance of skills between different facets. Although leadership and team working are similar in that they employ similar building blocks such as communication skills, they are in fact distinct and almost in conflict with each other—the leader leads, sometimes in a hierarchy with the buck stopping there, and the team worker is able to operate within a flatter hierarchy. You should be able to shift between these two positions and articulate that clearly, with a good understanding of your good and bad qualities and how these might contribute.

In this exercise, as well as facets, we might also consider aspects of ourselves that tend to express themselves during an interview, beyond our basic psychological states such as anxiety or excitement. Think about previous interviews and try to extract aspects of yourself that have become more prominent during social stressful interactions—you might also mine into other social experiences, such as first dates, parties, and public speaking. See past the anxiety and extract aspects of personality. A common aspect might be humour, another might be a shield of confidence. Use these aspects as examples, and try to find good and bad qualities that are relevant to these. Link them as above.

With your carefully and thoughtfully constructed list you can reflect on what you bring to the interview in a structured way. As a final step, circle the qualities, aspects, and facets that speak to your core values and beliefs. Which of these things speak passionately to you, and in turn can be presented passionately to the interviewer? Not too passionately though—always try to balance passion with detached professionalism. Just add a dusting of passion across your bedrock of professionalism and dissected aspects of personality and qualities.

Being mindfully anxious

It is normal and indeed essential to be anxious before a job interview. Being anxious allows us to perform to the best of our ability, giving us the adrenaline boost to power past any hiccups or awkward moments, and without anxiety we may appear flat or nonchalant. Interviews are exhausting, physically and emotionally, and our anxiety is like a physiological battery, powering us on in the face of adversity and stress. Also, this is a new chapter in life with fresh challenges and hurdles to overcome, a situation that demands our own sense of anxiety and perhaps one in which some anxiety might appropriately be communicated during the interview. Apart from anything, the interviewer expects you to be anxious, and whilst a lack of anxiety might on some level reassure them that you are up for the job, on the whole a lack of anxiety would probably make them worry. Do you really understand the level of skill and commitment required for this position? Are you ready for the responsibility?

We will consider anxiety in more detail later (see Chapter 6), but for now try to immerse yourself in the anxiety you hold for this interview, and let it perfuse into the skills and qualities you would potentially bring to the post. Anxiety feels unpleasant, it is uncomfortable, it can affect our sleep and strip away our enjoyment of life. Indeed, a lot of our time in life is spent trying to push ourselves into a state peace, away from the grittiness of anxiety—anxiety tells us that something is wrong. But in this situation, anxiety is important and should be mindfully embraced. Anxiety is our friend and ally in this interview process and we will nurture it, reframe it, and carry it with us at all times.

Why are we here?

This is a big question, and when the interviewer asks it I don't suggest that you launch into a lengthy existential narrative, but it is good to consider how this particular job fits into your life plan as a whole. A new job is a significant step in life and will take up a large amount of your time and resources—it is important, and it needs to complement life as a whole. How does this job do that? The honest answer might be that it provides you with the resources to do the bits of life you actually like, outside work, and we can all probably relate to that though we wouldn't say it in the interview. However, the interviewer is a person who knows there is a world outside the boundaries of this job, and it might be helpful to inject a flavour of what that looks like for you. If the interviewer expects you to work hard at the expense of the rest of your life perhaps this isn't the right job, or maybe you know that this is a period of time when your complete focus on work will have a massive impact on your future career trajectory. However this job fits into your life as a whole, it is worth reflecting on what it was that got you here and why you are sitting in this interview chair, with a wider perspective than just the job itself. Asking these difficult questions will give you a sense of inner resolution and purpose, and such resolution will probably be expressed to the interviewer even if you don't explicitly talk about the bigger issues at play. Just be honest, with yourself and with the interviewer, but also be mindful of how much they want and need to know—you are a cog in a wheel, you need to slot into place in this bigger machine and whilst your life narrative is important, just be aware of it and disseminate it only if directly asked. We know why we are here, that is all that matters.

CHAPTER 3

A framework of understanding

CONTENTS

Being mindful

Mindfulness is a key concept in modern psychiatric and psychological thinking, and an important process with many texts and books dedicated to it.[1] As busy humans we so rarely live just in the moment, instead finding ourselves thinking about the past or future, ruminating about things that could have been better, fantasizing about what might have been or might be. Being mindful is being grounded in the present; it is focussing on our breathing, our internal and external worlds, being present moment to moment as life unfolds around us. There is mounting evidence to suggest that a state of mindfulness is good for our physical and mental health[2], and it's probably worth developing this way of existing in all aspects of our lives. Perhaps you already have. Being mindful is a good skill to develop for the interview, and an excellent technique to employ in this psychologically loaded encounter. It is a way for us to remain focussed on exactly what's transpiring within this complex interchange of verbal and non-verbal communications, and not to lose ourselves in ruminations about what just went wrong or what questions might come next. All that matters is now, and all of our focus will remain grounded in the moment, where it's needed.

I have spoken in Chapter 2 about being *mindfully anxious* and we will consider that concept in greater detail later. In fact, mindfulness is in counterpoint to anxiety and is often used as way of reducing stress and anxiety. Anxiety tends to be rooted in either the future or the past—dread of what might come or rumination about what might have been, a sense that something isn't right. Mindfulness snaps us into the present moment, and without the echoes of the past or future worries clouding our perception of the world, it could be said that anxiety would not exist. Here and now, in this exact moment, breathing air and reflecting on our body and its connection to the world around us—the places our skin touches fabric, the colours and smells we experience, the sounds we hear just at the edge of our hearing—there is no anxiety. If we are able to dislocate ourselves from the echoes of the past and the future we can rid ourselves of anxiety, or at least reduce it. You have probably noticed anxiety-inducing tasks, such as night duty shifts or first dates, being marked by a prodromal anxiety that reduces significantly once you start the actual task— once you get on with it the anxiety melts away, and you are left with just the adrenaline initially associated with the anxiety. If you remain in an anxious state then you aren't really getting on with the task at all, you are just stuck in a position of contemplation. The difficulty with an interview is that the whole task is beset by a sense of contemplation—what will the next question be? What's the next hurdle to overcome? We need to mindfully exist purely in the task of the interview, and furthermore reframe contemplation during the interview itself. We will try to do that in this book.

There are many techniques available to us, to achieve a state of mindfulness, and perhaps you either know these already or might be feeling a desire to skip this section. I am not suggesting you start meditation or yoga, although both of these are fantastic ways of achieving a more mindful state of being. You probably find yourself slipping into more mindful moments, such as washing up crockery or gardening, cooking or bathing—these are moments in life when we tend to just exist in the moment, appreciating the world for what it is. At times of stress and mental poor health it is more difficult to remain connected to a task such as cooking and you might find your mind wandering towards the bills you need to pay or the chores you have left to do, rather that just feeling the food between your fingers and creating a nice meal for yourself and loved ones. Just as poor mental health tends to push us away from a state of grounded connection to the world around us and into an abstract space of fear and anxiety, if we pull ourselves back into the present moment and focus on the food as we prepare it our mental wellbeing will improve. Going through the interview process is not unlike going through any high stress period in life, a kind of self-inflicted mental insult, and pulling ourselves into the present will help us back towards a place of good health within the context of this psychological barrage of past and future echoes, underlying motives that we couldn't hope to understand, and nuances of communication that we simply can't fully grasp. We can use mindfulness to focus on the parts that are useful to us, here and now, and put to one side any psychological barriers or baggage that might otherwise hinder our performance in the interview.

As a starting point, try to develop your ability to concentrate wholly in the moment and do this by thinking only about your breathing. Feel the breath enter your body and fill up your lungs, reflect on the air as it leaves your body back out into the world. Right here, in this room, what can you hear? See? Smell? What are you touching? Is your skin touching just fabric clothing, or is part of your body in contact with wooden furniture? Just exist in this moment, not the past or the future, just right now. Think about the room, the fittings and fixtures, the colours and styles—don't dwell on what happened in this room yesterday or what might happen tomorrow, just exist here and now. Empty your mind of anything but the present and try to achieve this state daily for a short period of time, perhaps just 5–10 minutes. Try to achieve this state in different settings, perhaps a quiet room at work, a library, a swimming pool. Then try to achieve this state in more challenging settings, a busy café, a crowded book shop—just exist in the moment and focus your mind to the here and now. Do this daily and you will be building your strength, and sharpening your ability to focus your attention into the present space. You will then be more able to do this in your interview.

Motivations and expectations

The interview is a meeting of minds, an interchange of views, it is the establishment of a collaborative space that will be newly formed between you and the interviewer. You both exist in this collaborative space, trying to find a middle ground that might work in your new potential chapter in life. You both enter into this space with a set of motivations and expectations, and whilst it is impossible to know the extent of what is driving the interviewer, you can at least know exactly what is driving you. Why do you want this job? How will it change your life? What can you bring to the role? A standard opening interview question is something along the lines of 'please walk us through your CV and let us know the skills and qualities that make you the right person for this job'. Even if that question isn't explicitly asked, you need to know the answer to it before you walk into the room. You must also be aware of your own expectations, both of what is expected of you in the interview itself and subsequently if you were to be successful in gaining employment. You might expect to be treated with respect, to have a voice in the interview and the workplace, to have the possibility of an onward career trajectory. Try to reflect on your own motivations and expectations before the interview, have a good understanding of the pathway that led you to this point and where you expect that road to lead in the future.

As well as entering into this collaborative space with a clear understanding of our own motivations and expectations, let us now turn our attention to those of the interviewer. It is probably helpful to remember that whatever the level and type of employment, the interviewer will almost certainly be motivated by a desire to choose a candidate who is a person they could get on with, day-to-day, and one who would share basic ethical and core principles of both themselves personally and the company as a whole. Whatever is required in the actual post in terms of skills and attributes, the interviewer will probably expect you to be a diligent person who will take the roles and responsibilities inherent in this new post seriously. These conceptual motivations and expectations of the interviewer give us an access point to something important—how we can frame ourselves accordingly throughout, and furthermore how to package our anxiety away by focussing our attention onto the parts of the interviewer we can see and understand. The interviewer is a person who will have certain requirements for the human qualities in the person they employ. We shouldn't focus wholly on this, but it is a good starting point. When you sit down for your interview just remember that this interviewer, however intimidating, is just a human being and you should interact with them in a human way. Humans are not infallible robots, we are all fallible, liable to make mistakes and fluff our lines. We all sweat and stumble over acronyms, we all get dry throats and sometimes make mistakes. We don't need to be perfect, we just need to be us.

It's also worth considering what the role and purpose of this interview actually is. The job you are applying for is probably also sought by other worthy candidates, and since the essence of the interview process is one of competition, the interview is trying to push candidates to their limit in order to find areas of discrimination between them. If all the candidates just answered standardized questions in the same way then there would be nothing to distinguish between them. This is especially relevant in medical and surgical higher training interviews, where the trend is for a more standardized interview process with the questions often being published before the interview, available to all candidates, and the candidates often having very similar backgrounds and CVs. In this case it is even more important to score highly as a human being, since the boxes for the actual content are likely to be essentially ticked by all candidates. When the interview process is a more level playing field, the non-technical qualities you express as a person are even more critical as discriminators between you and others. You need to be the candidate who smiles, is relaxed and easy to be with, who can take something seriously but not too seriously, who is balanced and motivated without being arrogant or over-confident. You need to be consciously aware of your verbal and non-verbal body language, and how this will communicate the above to the interviewer, even though the questions are not explicitly asked. You need to measure and deliver yourself in the interview to cover all these bases, beyond the questions themselves, and in that way covertly answer some of the questions the interviewer has about motivation and expectation.

Much of this book speaks to how we might refine our non-technical dissemination of ourselves, but for now we will start with an exercise on refining our dissection and understanding of the environment of the interview (see Exercise 3.1 and Figure 3.1). We will learn to exist mindfully in the interview space, and provide the best possible template for our non-technical dissemination skills to be added to later.

This is an exercise that can be rehearsed every day, in any social situation you might find yourself in. The objective is to learn how to mindfully exist in a social space, being connected to the here-and-now, whilst also holding your attention in the external space of the room. It is so easy and potentially catastrophic to exist wholly inside ourselves during a stressful interview, thinking only about the answer we're giving, what we might say next, and what we already did wrong. Stress and anxiety tend to push us into an internal introspective space—here we will work towards moving out into the external space and thereby be examiners of the interview process from a more objective standpoint. We are remaining mindfully connected, we are undefended, and are mindfully anxious, but we are stepping out of our internal space and into the external room. Carefully and accurately reading the room is an excellent way of achieving this.

Take a piece of A4 paper and circle the word 'me' in the centre of the page (see Figure 3.1). This is our starting point, it is us, sitting here in the room, surrounded by the external world as it interfaces with our internal one. We will spend time elsewhere considering the inside of that circle, but for now we will devote ourselves to the things that surround us in the room. Draw three more circles around this one so that 'me' is the bull's-eye of a dartboard and the biggest circle fills the page—you now have three layers surrounding 'me' (see Figure 3.1). Label the first layer from the centre 'concrete', the second layer 'material', and the third layer 'abstract'. In any room we are surrounded at all times by these core elements.

Concrete objects are the table, chair, bookshelf, librarian, members of the public, a faded photograph—the actual things that surround us in this space. Material elements are also with us in this space: these are sounds, smells, textures, shadows, reflections, the ambient temperature—these are the sensory building blocks that underpin the concrete objects in the room and work with them to provide a scaffolding of elements that hold us here in the centre of this space. There are other things in this room with us, not just the concrete and material elements, but also abstract qualities that pervade through this space, instilling the objects and elements with meaning and providing a context that defines the atmosphere—such as a sense of oppression, a need for quiet, an angry librarian who keeps looking over at every turn of the page, a distracting person playing on his smart phone, the knowledge that the library will close soon, the fact that you are thirsty, perhaps you feel annoyed. Think about the space you are currently occupying and fill in the layers of concrete objects, material elements, and abstract qualities that surround you.

To explain the meaning of the concrete material and abstract a little further, imagine a lava lamp. The lava lamp itself is the concrete object. You switch it on and it emits light, a material element. It also might start to burn off some dust as the light heats up, the smell is another material element. The 'lava' moves as the lamp heats up—the lava is concrete, but the movement, the ebb and flow, is a material element. Once the concrete object of the lamp is emitting its material elements, the room appears more relaxed as the light and shapes perfuse the ambience of the space—this is an abstract quality of the lamp, i.e. the way it makes you feel. The lamp changes the atmosphere of the room, and this abstract quality infuses the lamp with a new identity—you know the lamp will create a relaxing atmosphere before you even switch it on, its abstract qualities perfuse even the inanimate concrete object when switched off. When switched on the object becomes a whole.

Now that you have written the concrete, material, and abstract qualities down, and have thereby constructed a written representation of the scaffolding that holds you here in the centre of this space, look at all the words and phrases on the page as they spread out from the centre and try to find links between them. Some links are obvious, such as the table feeling hard against your fingers, or the librarian giving you a sense of oppression. Perhaps the clock on the wall lets you know the room will close soon, and the member of the public is sitting too close and making you

(continued)

feel annoyed. Try to make links between the concrete, material, and abstract, and thereby build up a network of connections that start to make sense of these things that surround you in this space. Try to find some more obscure links between the concrete, material, and abstract. Perhaps you might suppose that the librarian is irritable because the room is too cold? Maybe their annoyance with you turning pages is making you feel oppressed and therefore making you less tolerant of the person on their smart phone? Try to link most of the words and phrases on the page beyond their own layer, and ideally link abstract things as far as you can. Indeed, the abstract things that surround us do tend to infuse everything with something that changes the context of the concrete and material. We will operate on this level in several different rooms and locations, and we will complete this exercise a few times a day—in that way, we will develop our ability to read a room in a concrete, material, and abstract way, and we will do this instinctually in the interview itself.

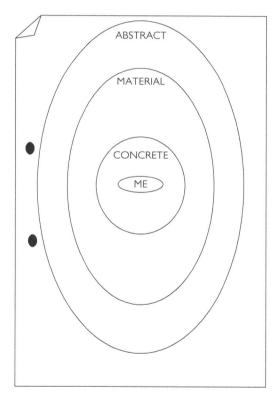

Figure 3.1 Reading the room
We are surrounded by concrete, material and abstract elements—make a note of those things around you using this template.

Being real

We have discussed authenticity and the importance of bringing your authentic self to the interview (see Chapter 2). We have spoken about building blocks of authenticity, and have thought about the way that these might be moulded into shapes that fit the expectations of the interviewer. We have considered the value of being authentic and truthful about ourselves as a people during the interview, in the same way we might at a first date, since this is the first page of a potential new chapter in our life and shouldn't just be a game or charade. Being real is being authentic, but here we will consider ourselves as being real in the interview room.

As soon as we enter the interview room we fill it with our concrete being, our material elements and also our abstract presence. Whilst an interview can feel like a process we are merely swept along in, and indeed we might be one of twenty candidates, during our twenty or so minutes the interview is all about us—we fill and change the interview space, we are the centre of attention. Later in this book we will use the concrete, material and abstract as ways of dissecting into our real being as we fill the interview space and will consider these components separately. For now, just consider the truth of your presence as you enter the interview room—this is about you, and everything you say and do has an impact in the room. Everything matters. Instead of just sitting down on the chair provided, move it slightly so you can sit more comfortably, and also so you assert your presence in the room. If there is a glass of water and you feel like it, take a sip. This is your time, your space, and you are a real being in this place. You matter.

Being real is also about being truthful and allowing yourself to be vulnerable. True strength is born from ones ability to embrace vulnerability, rather than denying weakness with a defence of external strength. Inside we are all vulnerable, and an interview pushes us further into a place of vulnerability. This can be uncomfortable and unsettling but it is important to recognize and embrace your vulnerability, and from there, find and disseminate true strength. If the interview questions go to a place that is more difficult, for example asking you to speak about times when things have gone wrong in the past or times when you have been in conflict with a colleague, embrace the challenge and answer from a truthful place of vulnerability. Truth in these questions will exude from every pore, as will any defence and lack of truth. A veneer of strength is unattractive when reflecting on such questions, it is much better to find strength within your vulnerability. For example, you may have been scared in a particular clinical situation, you may have acted precipitously—this should be carefully expressed but then you can find the strength within that act, such as explaining the subsequent process of supervision and reflection that allowed you to understand what went wrong and to reduce the chance of this happening again. Remember that future events are best predicted by historical ones—a true honest reflection would need to include the possibility that whatever went wrong could happen again, but that you are now aware of it. Being aware of the possibility of something going wrong is much more reassuring to the interviewer than a candidate in a fixed defended position of strength, operating under the illusion that it could never happen again. It might. This is true vulnerability, and this is being real.

Building the scaffolding

Now that we have conceptually broken down space into the concrete, the material and the abstract, including the part we play as real beings in that space, we can start to think about building our own scaffolding, our own construction to take with us into the interview space. We have, over the course of this chapter, found ways to break down and dissect into the world around us, so that we might be equipped with a framework of understanding that we can carry with us into the interview. Whether or not this framework is the absolute truth is inconsequential, indeed it isn't the truth since I have merely suggested this concept as a framework for the interview, but it is at the very least a new way to approach this stressful psychological experience. Change in itself is a good thing, in life and in the interview, and with this new perspective on the interview you will lose the psychological baggage perhaps collected in your previous interview experiences. Remember, psychological baggage is not just when things go wrong—baggage is also created when things go right. A brilliant prior interview can be just as much a burden as a disastrous one, since it is unlikely that whatever made the last one brilliant will recreate itself during this fresh new challenge in life. We should approach each interview with new eyes, a brand new perspective and page for a brand new chapter in life. Our new psychological framework of understanding will help us do this, and we will build upon this concept in detail later in this book.

References

1. Pagnini, F. and Philips, D. (2015) Being mindful about mindfulness. *Lancet Psychiatry*, **2**(**4**): 288–9.
2. Creswell, J. D. (2017) Mindfulness interventions. *Ann Rev Psychology*, **68**: 1–652.

CHAPTER 4

We all fail in interviews

CONTENTS

Moving on after failure

This may seem like a rather negative chapter in what I hope has been a positive book so far, and perhaps you might feel an urge to move on straight away. I would understand that, and in some ways it is not helpful to dwell on failures of the past, indeed I have spoken explicitly about being mindfully present and not existing in the past at all. However, learning from past mistakes is essential in this process, and the best lessons in life, and in the interview, are always made when things don't go well. Also, I would suggest that it's true to say that we all fail interviews, every single one of us. Even if all of our interviews have been successful in terms of getting the job, it must certainly be the case that we can all remember experiences that have tested us in the interview, and times when we have walked out of the room and felt we could have done better. Perhaps this isn't the case for you, but then perhaps you might not feel the need to read this book. Failure is all about threshold, and one person may feel a failure even if they do get the job, because they didn't do as well as they could do. For most of us, we will encounter at least one failure at interview, and perhaps more than one.

What is failure? What does it mean to you? Do you feel personally rejected by a lack of success? Are you able to hold the thought in mind you just weren't right for this particular job? I suggest that it is useful to consider failure in the interview as rejection—this might appear brutal, but now is not the time for ego-sparing fragile defences. Let us be frank, and accept the possibility that failure in the interview is actually rejection of us as a person. This will allow us to get the most out of our negative experience, both in terms of learning and personal growth. Being rejected is painful, whatever you are rejected by, and especially a job you feel you are right for and really want. Here we will think about ways to re-process failure into something that will help our next interview attempt, and find practical ways to learn from our mistakes. We should all approach an interview with a 'bring it on' attitude, so that we welcome things being tough since these will help to refine our skills and make us perform better in the future. To do that, we will start by embracing failure and accepting the painful fact that when it comes to the interview, we will all be rejected at some point and that we will all fail.

Another thing to consider, especially in this age of standardized medical interviews, is the slight edge one candidate can potentially have over another if they carry less psychological baggage into the process. A bad interview experience, or a previous rejection, can taint our performance unless we are able to carefully process the baggage and reframe it into something that fuels and potentiates our performance rather than hindering it. We need to learn from our mistakes and past failures, and with this new knowledge perform even better in the future. Unfortunately, these things can sit heavy on our shoulders and can put us in a slightly worse position than the next candidate who is free of such psychological burdens. We need to have all the edge we can get, especially if the distinguisher between candidates is not found within the content of the answers to interview questions, nor the quality of our CVs and prior experience. This book, and working through any negative interview experiences, will help you to develop an edge and help you to perform competitively, on a level playing field—to be the best you can be.

Grieving and acceptance

Rejection is painful especially when an interviewer rejects us for a job we really want, a job we think we are well suited to, and one that could take us forwards in life. Allowing ourselves to really want a job gives us the ability to shine in an interview and perform at our best, but it also allows the possibility of pain if we are unsuccessful. If we have failed in the past, and have not been successful when applying for jobs we really wanted and felt suited to, then we might find ourselves not really wanting jobs in the future—we might find ourselves numbed to the process with more of a take-it-or-leave-it attitude. This is normal, a normal defence protecting us from the potential exquisite pain of failure. To be successful we need to be open to the possibility of failure, we need to allow ourselves to really want a job and accept the truth that we may not be successful, it might be painful and it will probably take a while to get over. Every interview should be approached in this way, as an important formative experience that has the potential to be extremely painful, but one that could be life-changing if we were to be successful. We need to try to find that level of passion and bring it with us into the interview space. To do this, we need to truly connect with our failures, grieve our losses, and once that pain is felt and processed, move on to a position of acceptance.

Here, once again, mindfulness is a useful strategy. Mindfulness allows us to connect with the pain of failure, to soak in the uncomfortable water of rejection and allow it to wash through us. Connecting with failure and rejection gives us the valuable opportunity of asking the question 'why did I fail and why was I rejected?' If we dismiss the pain of failure then we are not able to fully process and understand it. I would suggest that the pain of failure is important, and if you don't feel pain with rejection and failure then you should question the psychological processes that took you into the interview and address them accordingly. Strip away the defences that are protecting you from this pain, don't allow yourself to be nonchalant about the prospect of this new chapter in life— embrace the excitement and possibilities that this new position might offer, and lose the mask of indifference that enables painless rejection as part of your journey. In the same way you connect with the present and with a room, connect with the possibility and actuality of failure.

Perhaps you are reading this and feeling detached from the words, detached from this pain, and maybe of the opinion that you are a positive person who is untouched by failure in this way. You might have been unsuccessful and found your own way of dealing with this, moving on, staying strong, and performing excellently in subsequent interviews. You might already possess interview resilience, and this wouldn't be surprising since we all have our own threshold and capacity for resilience. Some people let psychological adversity wash off them like water from a duck's back, it just doesn't stick. However, I suggest that as an interview gets more stressful, more challenging, and more important for a candidate, then the psychological processes and adversities get more 'sticky' and less easy to brush away. Moreover, even a person who is incredibly resilient in this process, with a high hit-rate of success, can still benefit from mining into the well of failure and rejection. Failure and rejection is a precious resource, and to utilize its potential we need to be able to process and move on after failure.

Let us consider failure as a process that we can utilize for our next interview—the following exercise may help with that (Exercise 4.1 and Figure 4.1).

EXERCISE 4.1 **UTILIZING FAILURE**

In order to move on after failure, we must first truly accept that we have failed. This is often difficult to do, since we have to get back to the day job and get on with the process of living. It is easy to blame interview failure on aspects of the process beyond our control, and often this might be the case. However, it is not useful to do only that, and even if it's true that the failure was born from things completely beyond our control, we need to work hard to find some gems and nuggets of failure that we can take ownership of, that are ours. We need to find and collect these precious stones, examine them carefully, and catalogue them away inside ready for our next interview.

Take a piece of A4 paper and divide it into three sections, with horizontal lines a third and two-thirds down the page (see Figure 4.1). Label the top section 'failure', the bottom section 'success', and the middle part 'moving forwards'. First think about an interview that went wrong, whether a total disaster resulting in failure or just an experience that could have been better, and write individual words in the upper 'failure' section capturing the main problem areas. These could be words such as 'anxious', 'awkward', 'I froze', 'the other was person better', and 'they already chose'. In this section, circle the words that are internal factors, i.e. to do with you, potentially under your control. External factors are equally important, just not circled here. Under each word in the upper section, write another word in red pen, representing how that word makes you feel now. So under 'awkward' you might write 'embarrassed'. Under 'they already chose' you might write 'annoyed'. Try to capture the main internal and external factors, as concisely as possible, and attribute a feeling to that factor.

Next, move to the bottom section of the page and write down words and phrases that capture the things you brought to the interview that could have potentially led to success in this job. It might be that you didn't properly express those things in the actual interview, e.g. perhaps you didn't demonstrate your confidence or skills properly because of anxiety; but list the assets you brought with you on the day. Examples might be words such as 'good communicator', 'team player', 'compassion', and 'good work ethic'. Circle the words you felt unable to fully demonstrate on the day, those areas that could have been better, and perhaps if they had been better you might have been successful. We won't neglect the other words, the assets you were able to successfully express—we just won't explicitly use them right now. Think about the assets and consider what it was that stopped you being able to properly express them. Was this similar in other interviews or just particular to this one? With a red pen, under each word or phrase capture how you currently feel when you think of this particular asset. You might find the emotions are tinged by whether or not the word is circled, i.e. a missed opportunity will induce sadness absent from the assets you were able to properly express in the interview.

Try to balance roughly the number of circled words in the upper and lower sections, but only try to do this—you need to capture your thoughts and feelings in these sections accurately, but just be aware that you are looking for a kind of rough equality. This is because we will be using the circled words in both of these sections to balance each other, and to find a way forwards. With this in mind, you may wish to circle more or less words in either or both of the sections. We are looking for a rough balance of weight between the internal factors that potentially led to failure, in the upper section, and the good parts of yourself that you were unable to properly

(continued)

express during the interview, in the lower section of the page. These things, the circled words, are critical for moving forwards. They are all within your locus of control, and they are the building blocks that will improve your future interview performance.

Now, with a green pen, you need to try to match a circled word in the upper section with one in the lower, and connect the circles with a green line. Match these words carefully, and match them only individually—a circled word in the upper will only link with one in the lower. You need to choose the best possible match and this decision should consider the following factors: similarity of focus or content, importance, critical nature, intensity, and the attributed current feeling. You are looking for circled words that match, but ideally the attributed feelings should also balance out in some way. For example, you might draw a line from 'awkward' in the upper section to 'good communicator' in the lower. These words are linked in that they are both critically important, and the awkwardness probably stopped you from communicating in the interview, ironically inhibiting a skill you brought to the interview. So your communication skills were inaccurately expressed during the interaction, despite what you might have said about them, because you were too awkward. You might have written embarrassed under 'awkward' and perhaps you wrote 'angry' under 'good communicator'. Balancing the current attributed emotions is not critical in this exercise, but reading them and thinking about them in this context is a useful adjunct. Also, so often do our thoughts become contaminated with emotion—by separately listing the attributed emotions we are packaging them separately, thereby decontaminating the thoughts.

Where the green lines pass though the middle 'moving forwards' section, write in black pen a short phrase by each line that captures both matched words as closely as possible, but frames the concept in an idealized way for the future. In the worked example above you might write 'speak slowly, be confident' across the line that joins 'awkward' and 'good communication'—you know you are a good communicator, you should feel confident about that, you just need to speak more slowly next time. You have moved forwards by deciding upon a strategy available to you, within your locus of control, that captures something that went wrong and also something that didn't reach its potential in the interview. In red pen, under the phrase, write the emotions you noted under the words individually earlier—these are your emotional anchors, pulling you back to the deconstructed psychological position from earlier. For success you need to retain these psychological building blocks, deconstructed facets of your potential failure and success, and hold this position alongside your newly constructed strategy for moving forwards. In this way, you are mindfully holding onto the pain of failure, whilst rebuilding this into something more positive for the future. You are not defending against failure and blindly floundering onwards—you are the investigator of your failure, mining down into your psyche, nurturing these precious stones, and furnishing yourself with a powerful set of pragmatic directions for your future performance.

Reframing loss into strength

Growth is an essential facet of human existence, and here we are concerned with our psychological growth and our development of resilience. Whilst we are constantly growing in a psychological sense, with every interaction and moment in life, experiencing loss pushes us into a state of vulnerability that enables significant psychological growth if we allow it. The old adage is: 'what doesn't kill us makes us stronger', a phrase I am sure we can all relate to. Don't brush the pain of loss aside, don't exist in a defended state away from failure and rejection—instead, embrace the pain of loss. Dissect into it, examine it, discuss it with a friend. Let the pain of loss soak through you, gently lower yourself into its depths. Don't deny loss, don't deny yourself this fantastic opportunity for growth. At the core of this, you need to accept the truth that you are good enough exactly as you are, and that this experience of loss, in the context of a failed interview, is a rare privilege. This

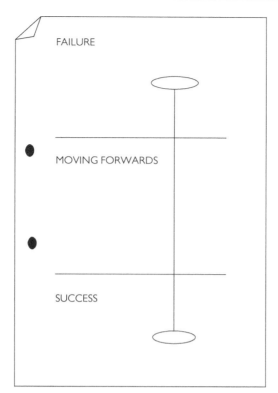

Figure 4.1 Utilizing failure
Accepting, breaking down, and reframing failure into something precious and useful for utilization in our future interviews.

is not the agonising loss of bereavement or the poor health of a loved one—this interview loss is something totally insignificant in the grand scheme of things. But although insignificant, the loss associated with failure in the interview is painful, perhaps more painful than it should be. Perhaps if we weren't in such a career-focussed world and society we really wouldn't care if we failed in an interview. But since we are in that world, embrace this opportunity to properly allow loss to diffuse through your mind and body, and thereby become stronger as a result. You are a psychological body builder, building strength and resilience as you allow the pain of loss to perfuse your muscles. Without the pain, there is no growth. Embrace the loss.

Failure within the interview itself

In some ways you can't fail until the interview is over, and we should all gain some comfort from that. How ever bad it's going, it can still be rescued. However, we can sometimes feel as though we've failed during the interview itself, and this negative mindset is rather like a self-fulfilling prophecy, enhancing the chance of failure. We might have not been able to answer a question, we might have interpreted the interviewer's shrug or yawn as indifference. There might have been a practical component to the interview that we messed up. Whatever the reason, it is essential to develop the ability to move on after our sense of failure within the interview itself, in order to give ourselves the best possible chance to pull things back from the brink. Indeed, we might have totally misread the interviewer's yawn, perhaps his child kept him up all night, and we might not actually have done that badly in earlier questions or tasks. We simply cannot allow ourselves the luxury of assuming we know exactly what the interviewer is thinking or how the interview has gone so far, since this is impossible. However we might assess ourselves, we have no idea how well other candidates have performed, and since the interview is at its heart a competitive process we must just exist in the moment and not dwell on those things over which we have no real knowledge and absolutely no control.

During a stressful interview there simply isn't time to recover naturally in the interview itself, to regroup and recover after something has gone wrong. Without a strategy to deal with this, such traumas during the interview can be potentially catastrophic for your subsequent performance. However, this realization in itself might give you some comfort, since it's exactly the same for everyone. Think about a time in life when a personal disaster has occurred, either inside or outside the interview—in personal disasters we have a tendency of attributing the problem wholly to ourselves, it is very difficult to reflect on the truth that most people would probably react in this way faced with similar adversity. Furthermore, stumbling over a question is actually a brilliant opportunity to demonstrate your resilience and your ability to bounce back to the interviewer. If something goes wrong, don't try to hide it or gloss over it—embrace it. We will think more later about how to physically embrace a disaster like this, and that might be something to do with a subtle shrug or a smile, literally shrugging the disaster off and moving on with the next question or task. See the disaster for exactly what it is—an opportunity for you to shine. Indeed, it may be the objective of the interviewer to push you to your limits in order to distinguish between you and the other candidates, and whilst it is unlikely that they would want you to trip up, if you do trip up they won't necessarily hold it against you. What is critical is how you manage to bounce back from the disaster, how you can gather yourself in front of their eyes and find the resilience to continue. With this, you are literally showing them your capacity to accept your own limitations and that you can move past these.

Another technique is to develop the ability to focus wholly in the moment, and we have spoken about that at length already in this book. If something goes wrong you shouldn't dwell on it, you need to move on, and actually you need to move from an internal position of rumination to an external position. Exist externally, in the interview space and focus your attention into the room, the interviewer, what is on the desk, the expressions of the others in the room, etcetera. Exist mindfully in the present and think about the concrete, material, and abstract elements in the room. Breathe. Consider how you are interacting with the elements in the room, how your physical presence changes the balance in the room, and move your focus away from inside your head—you don't have the luxury of being able to dwell inside right now, you need to be present outside instead. Use Exercise 3.1: Reading the room (Chapter 3), as a psychological method to move away from the disaster and back into the room.

Shifting perspectives

A common theme in this book is the idea of stepping outside of ourselves in the interview, being more present in the external space and less preoccupied by our internal thoughts and ruminations. To do this, we need to shift our perspective from internal to external, and at various points in this text I will suggest strategies of achieving this. So far in this chapter I have alluded to the simple fact that failure in the interview process is actually an opportunity to demonstrate resilience, both internally after the interview is over, and externally to the interviewer during the interview itself. Failure is an opportunity for growth and development, it is an opportunity for change. These things should start to help shift your perspective on failure, and whilst you may always wish to be successful, I hope that failure is something you can recognize as both essential for this process and something that should be embraced rather than dismissed. We have also considered shifting our focus from an internal space to an external one, and we have learnt some skills and techniques to help us do this in real time during the interview itself. In finally addressing failure, I suggest that your perspective should shift a little further still, not into the mind of the interviewer but into the mind of your future self, a future version of you who was successful in getting the job and is now giving the present version of you advice and guidance. What would you say to yourself? What advice would you give? Imagine yourself exactly where you wish to be, fill that space and embody it with all your unlocked hopes and aspirations, no longer shackled by the numbing defence of protection from the pain of failure. Allow yourself to be in that precious place, however fragile a fantasy that might be, and guide yourself though this difficult process. Be your own self-fulfilling prophecy. You deserve it.

Being connected

CONTENTS

The value of empathy

Being connected to the interview process as a whole, and the interviewer in particular, is essential. Stress and anxiety during an important interview will tend to push us to a more detached intellectual position, but for success we must retain our ability to connect with our emotions rather than being mindlessly driven by them. The way we stay connected during the interview, both to the interviewer and to our underlying emotional state, is by nurturing and utilizing our empathy. Empathy is about being human. Empathy is the way we connect with the world around us, the way we read others, and the way we express ourselves. In the real world, over a coffee with a friend or loved one, empathy is natural for most of us—it is effortless and normal. A moment of empathic silence when a friend breaks bad news, a small shake of the head and a gentle request to ask if they are okay is quite normal and authentic. Empathy is our currency in social communication, some of us are perhaps richer than others but we can all make this basic human trade, and we all must as part of a structured civilized society. Empathy is not just about what you say, or the way you say it— it is when you say it, why you say it, and what other non-verbal communications are made as you say it. Empathy has weight—an empathic communication, whether verbal or non-verbal, is driven by something beyond the external, and reflects underlying care, mutual respect, and understanding.

Whilst societal empathy is natural and easy to establish, empathy in an interview is not so easy yet just as important. Critical even. Empathy in an interview lets the interviewer know you are human, it lets them know that you care and that you would be a good person to work with. Empathy in the interview engenders your presence in the room with a sense of mutual respect and understanding. It allows you to express underlying emotions in a subtle way, enabling you to express yourself in a more nuanced way. Empathy is a social communication that cuts through all the noise of an interview, it cuts through the content and pragmatics of the questions and gets straight to the heart of the interviewer. Being empathic is essential, but in the heat of the moment will be hard to achieve—unlike a coffee with a friend, you will be less able to fall back on instinct and intuition. During an interview, especially one that pushes you to the limits of your abilities, passive instinctual skills such as empathy will be the first to disappear. With all your attention directed at answers to questions you will have less capacity to connect empathically, but to do so is essential—instilling your interaction with empathy will improve the quality of your communication and express so much more than what you overtly say and do. Your empathy needs to be refined and applied, like any other non-technical skill in the interview. In this chapter we will do that.

First let us consider empathy as a skill, and find ways of utilizing it as such in the interview—the following exercise will get us started (Exercise 5.1 and Figure 5.1).

EXERCISE 5.1 UTILIZING EMPATHY AS A SKILL

We start under the shared assumption that empathy is a powerful skill essential for your best possible interview performance. Some candidates will find it easy to empathize in the interview, whether because they are just naturally gifted that way or that this particular interview is not such an intellectual challenge for them. For most of us, in a stressful interview, we will lose our innate instinctual ability to connect empathically because we'll be concentrating too hard on the task at hand. This exercise will teach you how to distil, extract, and develop key empathic skills that you can then deliberately apply during your interview, thereby levelling the playing field between you and the candidate who can empathize with ease, and putting you in a good position to enable your best possible interview performance.

Actors employ empathy in high-pressure situations all the time—indeed, a performance lacking empathy appears drab and inauthentic. For this exercise we will observe, catalogue, and break down empathic moments, both those that we experience ourselves in real life and those that we watch performed by actors.

Take an A4 page and divide it into an upper and lower section with one horizontal line across the middle (see Figure 5.1). At the top of the page capture an empathic moment between two people, either one you've witnessed or one that you were party to—write the moment down in a sentence, with enough detail so that you can recall it exactly. Divide the upper section of the page into three columns with two vertical lines. Label the first column 'facts', the second 'thoughts', and the third 'feelings'. In the first column list all the facts associated with the empathic moment, for example: the setting, the intent of the interaction, the motivations driving the interaction, the outcome. In the second column list the distinct thoughts you had whilst watching or experiencing this interaction, such as: one person is right, you agree with a certain perspective, you would do or say things differently, this could have been a shorter or longer interaction. In the third column write down the feelings that were invoked in you whilst watching or experiencing the encounter, such as: anger, sadness, frustration, hope.

Next, consider the words and phrases in each of the columns and try to find links between them, ideally linking different columns together. For example, you might draw a line between the motivations of the two people and anger, or find a link between your sense that the interaction could have been longer, with frustration. Do the same with other empathic moments, using a new page for each and filling the upper section—break the empathic interactions down into the components of fact, thoughts, and feelings, and link as many as you can.

Breaking down the empathy into separate components allows us to examine the individual elements that give the moment power, and to consider which of those elements are most critical for its overall impact. It might be that the underlying motivations of the characters, plus the feeling of anger or urgency, are the most critical elements for a particular scene or experience. Think about the empathic moment and circle the words or phrases that are most critical in giving the moment power—without these circled elements, the empathy would be lost. An important element to many empathic interactions is compassion—really caring about something, whether expressed in a positive or negative way, tends to give a moment an emotional punch. What are the underlying emotions driving this empathic moment? Add words to the columns if you need, make a note of any underlying emotions in red pen to distinguish them from your existing elements.

(continued)

EXERCISE 5.1 (CONTINUED)

In the lower half of each page think of an interview question, relevant for your upcoming interview, and linked as closely as possible to the content of the empathic interaction that you have written down. Write the question at the top of the lower section of the page, and choose a question that might be acted with the same empathic drive as the moment above. The content linking the question to that empathic moment is not necessarily linked to what exactly was said in that moment, but perhaps the feelings or thoughts might be linked in some way. For example, a charged empathic moment between two characters in a courtroom drama, where one asks the other why they did what they did, might translate to a potential interview question about why you might want that particular job. The empathic acting could include passion of conviction, real emotion, and authenticity—and whilst you won't act to that extent in the interview, you have at least dissected into an extreme version of such an empathic exchange. Separate the lower section into three columns and label them fact, thoughts, and feelings. List the elements, the facts, thoughts, and feelings, you think might be relevant for this interview question if it were to be transposed into the empathic moment detailed above. For example, write down the empathic building blocks, the facts, thoughts, and feelings, for the interview question about why you might want this job, and transpose that into the same question being asked in that courtroom scene. Instil the question with those elements that would give the question an emotional punch so that it would fit into the scene above. Circle the most critical elements, those that are needed for the empathic punch—these are likely to be similar to the critical elements in the example above.

When you rehearse interview questions, think about the empathic punch of your responses and apply them in a subtle way. If the punch is delivered by having a true passion for the job, then deliver that subtly when you rehearse answering the question. Apply the empathy deliberately, and consider the elements you are employing in that process—the facts, the thoughts, and the feelings. Ask your rehearsal partner how they felt when you answered their question. Think about the building blocks of empathy when they answer your questions. Analyse and apply empathy as a skill, and hold in mind the broken down elements alongside the overall impression and emotional punch. This is a fine balance, and with practice you will be more able to apply empathy deliberately when you need to. In your interview, when you are potentially anxious and stressed, you can then answer the question about why you want the job in a way that will mean something more to you and the interviewer. You can add emotional weight to your responses, even at times in the interview when you simply don't have the capacity to connect with your underlying emotions in an instinctual way. Instead, act.

Emotional weight

Emotional weight is the driving force behind an empathic connection with another person, it is the engine powering our human communication. You should be aware of the emotions that power your answers to questions during the interview, and be mindful of the way these might come across. On the whole, we will concern ourselves here with trying to distil our emotions into something useful in the interview, as powerful engines to drive us forward in the process in order to communicate effectively and empathically. We will dissect out our emotions, linked to empathic skills, and apply these deliberately at key points during the interview. Exercise 5.1 will help you to do that.

However, for answers to include emotional weight it is not necessarily the case that you need to speak whilst being emotional—indeed, to do so could be a mistake. Emotion can sometimes distort our responses in the wrong way, if we are too emotionally connected to the question or concept. If we are emotionally overwhelmed then the objective here might be to strip out some

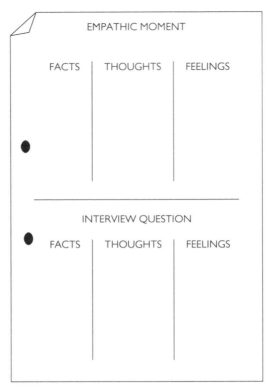

Figure 5.1 Utilizing empathy as a skill
Distil, extract, and develop key empathic skills.

of the emotion driving our natural empathy. For example, it is never attractive to want something too much, and no answer should be driven by a sense of desperation or neediness. Empathy driven by emotion should be applied with care in an interview, and whilst it might sometimes be very powerful to add a sprinkling of genuine instinctual empathy, even this should be done deliberately. Consider also that being too empathic in a work situation can potentially lead to burn out, so it is worthwhile to keep any overt emotions in check. However, thinking about the emotions that drive particular aspects of the interview—the questions asked, the potential answers, and the motivations behind these—is a useful exercise in itself. Being more aware of the emotional weight, both from yourself and the interviewer, is helpful for you in order to understand what unsaid factors are at play in the room.

Whilst you should do so with care, there are certain times when you should try to apply emotional weight to an answer. Like empathy, this might normally happen naturally but in the interview we simply cannot rely on normal instinctual mechanisms, we need to apply emotional weight deliberately. Anxiety will tend to numb our natural emotional responses, leaving us as intellectual shells in the interview, answering from our head and not necessarily engaging our heart. But some answers do require the contribution of one's heart, and whilst you shouldn't be driven merely by the superficial emotions present in your anxious state, you should take a deep breath and tap into the core emotions driving that particular aspect of the interview. Don't be a slave to your sense of urgency and neediness, don't be driven by the overpowering emotion that you really need this job. Instead, take a moment to reflect, and mine down to the emotion that drove you along this pathway in the first place—a sense of hope for patients in this particular field or community, a feeling of hope that you might be able to contribute to this area in a meaningful way. These are the emotions you need to get to, to fuel your empathic connection in the interview. Just be mindful of what your emotions actually are, and choose to focus on the ones that will drive your interview in a positive, truthful, and authentic way.

A shift in perspective

Let us once again consider a shift in perspective, from the internal space out into the external space of the interview. In this case, we will step out of ourselves and see the interaction through the eyes of the interviewer. Aside from rehearsal and consideration of empathy and the emotional weight that drives it, how else can we apply empathy as a skill in the interview? Often we will find ourselves stretched to capacity with the intellectual challenges an interview can pose, and we will probably be applying all of our resources to the questions and answers themselves. As I have said, and I hope you already agree, applying a sprinkling of empathy alongside your well thought out answer can only help the situation, and will allow you to connect with the interviewer or panel in a more human way. Herein lies the key to applying empathy, even in the intellectually toughest of situations—we are all human, both interviewees and interviewers. It's an obvious comment and I do not want to appear condescending, but in my own field of adolescent forensic psychiatry it is incredibly helpful to remind myself that we are all human. Criminals, like us and the interviewer, have human feelings and emotions, and are driven emotionally in the ways they interact. Even if emotions are skewed, or if the interviewer is exhausted and has absolutely no capacity left to connect with us as human beings, they are still human. In the interview, especially if it is a tough one, try to put yourselves into the shoes of the interviewer. See yourself through their eyes. When they ask a question take a moment to reflect on the situation from their perspective—not just the question itself, but the whole situation. The room, the other panel members, the other candidates, the job in question—put yourself into their mind as best you can, and thereby add some theoretical context to the questions they ask. You are not trying to answer in the way they want, instead you are authentically answering but with a more objective contextual standpoint, one that tries to incorporate their position as well as your own. After all, an interview is a meeting of minds, a collaboration of intent. By shifting perspective slightly you will be more able to empathically and emotionally connect with the moment, as you will be stepping outside of your own anxieties and baggage, and viewing the interaction from a more objective standpoint. If you see the human in them, they will be more able to see the human in you.

Speech, body language, and facial expression

Empathy is not so much what you say, although the words are important—it is more the way you say it, the way you come across. It is not about explicitly expressing that a statement has emotional weight, it is about implying that in a subtle way through your inflexion in speech, the tone of your voice, and your body language. Sometimes a more detached intellectual standpoint is appropriate, and in that case you would dial back the emotion—but the realization of that fact and your deliberate dialling back of emotion also employs empathy. Empathy is our understanding of the underlying unsaid components of an interaction, and sometimes you might appropriately choose to appear less emotionally empathic. This is similar to seeing a patient, connecting with their distress and pain with a warm empathic approach, and then choosing to pull back to a more paternalistic standpoint when you discuss treatment options—we change our standpoint depending on the needs of the social interaction. In this example, you might find yourself empathizing with the patient as they discuss their worries and concerns with a soft gentle voice, matching their own volume, and your body language might be more relaxed with a caring frown. But when you wish to pull the patient back to a more professional, positive objective standpoint, and you wish to inject the interaction with a sense of hope, you might speak in a gentle but clearer tone, with slightly higher volume, and you might straighten your body and appear more relaxed and confident in your facial expression. In this way, you are subtly pulling the patient back to a more objective and hopeful standpoint, literally pulling them out of the pain you were just sharing with them moments before. This is an example of the subtleties of empathic communication, and how we can apply speech, body language, and facial expression as a tool to accompany our social communication skillset.

Regarding speech, to be empathic we must be overtly in control of our tone and cadences, instilling the interviewer with confidence that we are relaxed and ready for this new position. True authentic instinctual empathy is born from a sense of relaxed calm, but we cannot rely on being able to access that state during the interview. Indeed, we need to be operating in a more heightened state, reading the room and being entirely present, fielding questions, and interacting in this critical process to the best of our abilities. We must apply empathy deliberately, and the biggest 'tell' of our internal state of calm is the nature of our voice. It is okay if you are so nervous that your voice initially breaks and perhaps you need to centre yourself by drinking some water, but you should be aiming for a volume of speech that is matched to that of the interviewer, and a tone that implies warmth and relaxation. If the interviewer speaks more quietly then subtly match that. Likewise, if they increase in volume you can too. Try to rehearse this every day: during those stressful interactions when you might otherwise race ahead or speak loudly, instead pull yourself back to a tonic level of calm and control. The volume and tone of your voice can have a powerful, calming, and containing influence on those around you, and you should deliberately employ this during your interview.

Body language is critical during an interview, and whilst it is obvious that one should not express their internal turmoil and anxiety by wringing fingers or rocking in the chair, getting in control of one's body language can be a struggle during a stressful interview. A good way to tackle this is to accept the importance of body language as a component of your empathic unsaid communication with the interviewer and apply this deliberately just as you apply other components. In that way, taming your body language is no longer just about how you feel and your internal world—it is actually about the way you are interacting in a socially nuanced way with another person. The interview is a collaboration, and your body language contributes to what is actually happening in the interview room—just as you might find yourself acutely aware of the interviewer fiddling with their pen, or a squeaking gutter just outside the window, the interviewer will be acutely aware of your finger squeezing. Be aware of your body language and present an external image of quiet controlled inner calm. Do this deliberately, and modify your posture as the situation warrants—if you are asked an especially challenging question then your body language should react accordingly, and rather than sitting stock still in the chair you might raise your hand to your chin or nod pensively while you think for a moment. Your body language is an extension of whatever else is going on inside—but rather than being a truthful 'tell' about your internal anxiety and turmoil, it should be an applied 'tell' that reinforces their impression of your calm authority.

Like our speech and body language, facial expression is a powerful indicator of our true internal state. Whilst we aspire to be truly calm internally during the interview, if we really were truly calm then we're probably not being pushed to our proper limits. Instead, our tonic internal state will be one of mindful anxiety, but such a truth could potentially give the interviewer the wrong impression. Our face should be relaxed at all times unless we want to specifically use it to reinforce our applied empathy, and if we are asked a challenging question then our face might appear pensive whilst we carefully consider our answer. We might express a range of emotions during the interview, but if we feel passionately about a particular job perhaps the best way of expressing that passion is via our face, alongside a more objective, professional, narrative. We might express sadness, and if asked to consider these times of austerity and the potential cuts over the next five years, our face would be a good way of communicating this, whilst our narrative might prefer to be more positive, utilizing the stretched resources as a passenger for change and optimization of services. Being detached and dispassionate during an interview is not a good thing, but without some due consideration on your facial expression you might find that interview stress and anxiety push your face flatter than it normally would be, giving the impression of emotional detachment. Practise moving your face, as a way of expressing your emotions, and apply this skill during your interview. In that way you will appear more thoughtful and empathic to the interviewer.

For all of these facets of empathy, it might be useful to video yourself during rehearsal. We will consider that in more detail later in this book (see Chapter 9).

Further reading

Harding, D. (2014) 'Forming a connection', in *Deconstructing the OCSE*. Oxford University Press, Oxford.

CHAPTER 6

Stress and anxiety

CONTENTS

The value of anxiety

Anxiety is a precious commodity in the interview, and rather than trying to stifle or dampen it down to a more comfortable state of relaxed internal calm, we should examine our anxiety, nurture it, reframe it into something that will overtly help. We should control our anxiety rather than letting it control us. Anxiety can be our ally in this process, and since it will be with us in some capacity whether we like it or not, we may as well use it to our advantage. Anxiety can feel unpleasant and we spend much of our lives trying to negotiate a world around us that keeps any anxiety at an absolute minimum, whether with our supportive network of understanding friends and colleagues, or by choosing a career pathway in life we can easily cope with. It might be that your ideal job would lead to more anxiety in life, and perhaps that's a sacrifice you're willing to take for the sake of improved income or increased esteem. Perhaps in this case, a lack of money or esteem leads to an overall life burden of anxiety for you that will be redressed by taking a hit of an increased level of work-specific anxiety? Or maybe you crave the increased pressure? In some ways, progression through life inevitably leads to an increase in anxiety, whether by increasing responsibilities at work or building a family who might depend on our successes. But even if your ideal job would ultimately lead to a reduction in anxiety, it is safe to say that for all of us, the interview is a period of anxiety that we must pass through in order to fulfil our aspirations.

Although anxiety can feel uncomfortable, it also pushes us into a state of increased efficiency, flooding us with adrenaline and optimizing our performance. An interview candidate lacking anxiety will probably be at a slight disadvantage to an anxious candidate, since the adrenaline on board the anxious candidate will drive them forwards to perform better. However, anxiety can go too far and push us into a place where we are less able to perform our best; anxiety can flood us with negative cognitions and can paralyse our instincts and natural responses. Anxiety can push us into a more defensive intellectual position and cut us off from our underlying feelings and emotions, those nebulous things that are so important to us in the interview. In this chapter we will reflect on our anxiety and work towards keeping it in check, reframing it into the positive psychological driver it can be, and protecting ourselves from any paralysing anxious overload. Here, we will actively choose to be *mindfully anxious*.

Reframing anxiety

Anxiety is a feeling, a mood-state, a nebulous sense that perhaps something is wrong, that something needs to change—but it stems from underlying thoughts and cognitions that can be easily accessed. Before we can reframe anxiety into a useful force for good, we need to understand it. At the time of feeling anxious it is often difficult to identify what led us to that anxious state, but more often than not, with some time and effort the triggering thought or event can be easily identified. Whilst it might be the case that in the days and weeks before an interview we feel generally more anxious, certain thoughts or events will probably trigger us and make us feel worse. It is worth trying to investigate the causes and triggers for your own pre-interview anxiety, because by doing so you will gain a deeper understanding of the factors that can potentially destabilize your composure, and you will be more able to keep anxiety in check during the interview itself. One way to do this is to keep a mood diary—a daily record of your mood-state, with notes detailing the events and thoughts that occurred around the time of the onset of anxiety. When you feel anxious, or indeed when you feel any strong emotion or mood, whether it be happy or sad, angry or frustrated, make a note of the date, time, and capture the emotion as closely as possible. Next to this, make a note of the thoughts that are going through your mind and try to identify the most prominent thought. After this, make a note of something in the external environment that can bring you back to this moment, whether it be a detail about the location or perhaps a mention of the people around you. If you do this consistently over a few days, and then re-analyse the statements at a time when you are no longer experiencing that particular mood-state, then patterns will start to emerge. You might find that particular thoughts lead directly to anxiety. But like anything in life, investigation in itself can change the nature of whatever is investigated, and with examination into your own mood-state you might find your anxiety starting to shift. At the very least, you will have a greater appreciation of the kind of thoughts and events that lead you to feel anxious.

An interesting aspect of anxiety is that often the underlying thought or cognitive process that makes us feel anxious can actually be reinforced and entrenched by our own actions to reduce the anxiety. This is an important concept, and appreciation of this in itself can be very helpful in reframing anxiety. An example of this is my own experience of being mugged: I felt justifiably anxious after this traumatic event and started to take the bus home rather than walking. Taking the bus reduced my anxiety, but it also reinforced the underlying belief that if I walked I would be mugged again. When I realized this, I decided to walk home—when I reached the place I had been mugged I was incredibly anxious, but as I walked past that spot I felt my anxiety literally lift away from my shoulders. In walking home I challenged the underlying belief that I would be mugged again, and provided powerful evidence to the contrary. What are you anxious about in the days and weeks before your interview? It is likely that your anxiety is at least partly driven by an underlying belief, such as the belief that you will fail or will say the wrong thing. If you have ways in life to reduce your anxiety, such as distracting yourself with music or television, or maybe having a drink of alcohol, then although your anxiety will reduce in the short-term you might inadvertently be reinforcing an underlying belief or cognition. Also, dampening down anxiety before the interview will tend to give it free reign to emerge triumphantly during the interview itself, whereas examining your anxiety will help to keep it in check. As a general rule, I would suggest that you try to sit with your anxiety, and instead of pushing it away and dampening it down, try instead to exist in that uncomfortable state and examine the thoughts and underlying beliefs that push you into this place.

The next phase in reframing anxiety, after examining your associated thoughts and considering your underlying beliefs, is to embrace this driving force for exactly what it is: physiological and psychological fuel for your interview. Consider a weight lifter who works hard in the gym—his muscle pain as he lifts weights is analogous to your sense of anxiety. The weight lifter knows that without the muscle pain, he is not building muscle, and he will push himself until he feels that burn.

Interview anxiety is not just a normal and expected part of this process—it is also a necessary component. As well as this, from your perspective, anxiety is one of the elements present in the room during the interview, as present as a draft from the window or noise from the street outside. Rather than trying to stifle and deny its existence, embrace it and take it on board as a necessary companion in this process. Being curious about one's own anxiety in an anxiety-provoking situation like an interview can be a very worthwhile exercise. Often our anxiety will give us a good indication as to what is actually happening in the room, it's our primitive inbuilt surveillance system and can provide us with information about not only our own internal state, but also with knowledge about the complex social dynamics that are occurring around us. This thinking is along the lines of the concept of counter-transference in a therapeutic interaction—how a social dynamic and interaction actually makes us feel can give us very useful information about the nature of that complex dynamic, if we are able to listen to and take note of our own feelings. Here, we will try to listen to our anxiety, take note of it, and be mindfully anxious.

In this next exercise we will work together to monitor, investigate, and understand our anxiety, with the objective of becoming mindfully anxious (Exercise 6.1).

EXERCISE 6.1 BEING MINDFULLY ANXIOUS

In an interview book like this one, you might have expected a chapter on anxiety that teaches you how to reduce anxiety, to be more relaxed, with an exercise on relaxation techniques. Not here. If a person has psychological help for anxiety they might be taught relaxation techniques, and these can be very powerful. However, if a person seeks help for an anxiety that leads to changes in their behaviour, for example, anxious obsessive thoughts that lead to compulsive behaviours that only ritualized compulsive behaviours will abate, then the psychological therapy is very different. In this more extreme case of anxiety, the therapeutic approach is the opposite of relaxation, it is instead about accepting and sitting with the anxiety whilst acting in a way that actually induces the anxiety. We will be approaching anxiety from this second position—not because our anxiety is so extreme that it needs a more extreme approach, but because in the interview anxiety tends to modify our actions and behaviours; and also because interview anxiety will not just drift away, it is a necessary part of the process and is here to stay. This exercise is built upon the premise that anxiety is necessary and inevitably present, and rather than denying or stifling it, anxiety should be examined, nurtured, and embraced.

Here we will keep a diary over the course of a few weeks, and we will make a note of times in our life when we feel anxious. This is a mood diary, and we will also note times when we feel especially happy, or angry, or indeed any powerful emotion. Finding the threshold of when to make a note of these emotional experiences will depend on you—I would suggest aiming to make two or three entries a day, so set the threshold at around there. It will take a few days before you get the balance right. Prioritize feelings of anxiety and have a lower threshold for detailing these than the other emotions, but it is important to balance the anxiety with a record of your entire emotional palate. Each emotion recorded should be on a separate diary page.

At the top of each page make a note of the date, time of day, where you were and what you were doing at the time of the emotion. Under this, note the emotion, e.g. anxiety, and try to record the emotional intensity as a score out of ten. Under the emotion divide the page into three columns and label them 'thoughts', 'facts', and 'consequences'. In the first column try to identify the prominent thoughts present during, and ideally just before, the anxiety—circle the most prominent thought, the one most likely to have triggered the anxiety. In the next column list the contextual factors relevant for that moment—these are the actual objects or people around you, or could be the things that were said at that time. You might list specific objects that can take you back to the

(continued)

EXERCISE 6.1 (CONTINUED)

feelings, e.g. objects on the table if you felt anxious over dinner, or the content of the conversation you were having just before and during the feeling. In the final column list the consequences of your feeling anxious—these might be your physiological response, e.g. feeling nausea, or could include a thought process triggered by your sense of unease. Consequences might also include your actions, i.e. what you actually did as a result of the anxiety. In this final column circle the most significant consequence that led to a reduction in your anxiety state—it is normal that anxiety will induce behaviour in us to reduce the anxiety, and these might be things such as distraction techniques or drinking alcohol. Try to identify the things you do to reduce anxiety.

This is your mood diary, and it is very difficult to properly assess and pull all this information apart when you are still feeling anxious. However, it is much easier to reflect on all these elements after the event, perhaps a few days later, when you no longer feel anxious. Read through your mood diary entry when you feel calm, and try to remember how the trigger thought made you feel, try to remember how the consequential behaviour acted to reduce your anxiety. Mentalize, i.e. think about the processes that were occurring when you were anxious—be curious about the anxiety, and investigate your own emotional state. Keep a diary over a few weeks and patterns will start to form—trigger thoughts will start to jump out, as will behavioural consequences that act to reduce your anxiety. Investigating these patterns is in itself useful—in this way you will start to spot anxiety before it hits, and will have a deeper understanding and knowledge of your mood state alongside your anxiety-reducing behaviours.

The next step in this exercise, after you have identified behaviours that act to reduce your anxiety, is to *stop* those behaviours. Here, instead of stifling and dismissing anxiety, we will be curious and will sit within our anxious state. Any action you might normally do to reduce anxiety should be stifled and dismissed, since these actions may well be reinforcing underlying beliefs and cognitions that actually fuel the mood state. But even if they aren't, here we are interested in being at one with our anxiety, welcoming it into our lives like a friend and sitting with it, at least for a while. I recommend sitting with your anxiety for at least ten minutes, letting it flow through you, and allow yourself to connect with the sensation and experience. Surrender to your anxiety, do not fear it—welcome it. If you can, use your mood diary to induce a state of anxiety—study the trigger thoughts and try to let them lead you to a more anxious place. Then sit with the anxiety and disregard any normal patterns of anxiety-reducing thoughts or behaviours. Allow yourself to be mindfully anxious.

The final part of this exercise can only be executed once you have allowed yourself to sit with your anxiety for ten or so minutes, and then, rather than distracting yourself or drinking alcohol to feel better, instead you will perform a body scan. A body scan will allow you to localize your anxiety, and with this basic technique you will work towards defining and visualizing this unpleasant feeling.

After allowing yourself to feel anxious for ten minutes, lie or sit back and close your eyes. Concentrate on your breathing, and keep the breaths steady and constant, in and out. Feel the breath go into your lungs and stomach, be nurtured and fed by the oxygen. Next concentrate on your toes, then work slowly up to your feet and ankles, calves, thighs, buttocks, lower back, and upper back, etcetera. Focus on each part of your body in turn and be curious about what you find there. Often we feel anxiety localized in our chest or neck, as a sense of tightness or pressure. Sometimes anxiety is found in the mouth or head. When you find an area of tightness, examine it, think about it—in this way you are examining the anxiety as an external entity, rather than it being an integral part of you. Don't reject or fear your anxiety, sit with it and try to imagine what it looks like. Try to assign a colour to it. If it is black, don't try to erase it—instead, flood that area of blackness with warm white light, smother the anxiety with a feeling of compassion. Identifying, localizing, and visualizing the anxiety will change its nature—you will notice that straight away. This is being mindfully anxious, and with this technique your anxiety will come to be a useful ally in your interview.

Understanding and utilizing stress

Just as we cannot deny and smother our anxiety in the interview process, we also cannot defend against stress. Stress is an essential component to the interview, and whilst the interview process tries to reduce undue stress for the candidates since it is in no one's interest to have stressed candidates, it is an unfortunate fact that this process is a stressful one. Stress on anything in life pushes the object to the limits of what it can take, whether it be a wooden scaffolding taking the weight of bricks, or you in the days and weeks before an interview. Life is already hard enough, so adding any further pressure will inevitably start to cause stress, and will start to push you towards the limits of endurance. Stress can be overwhelming, but alongside this it also gives us a strong sense of meaning and purpose—stress is absolute concrete proof that we matter in the world. Being pushed to the limits of endurance also gives us the opportunity to prove to the world where those limits are, to prove how much we can take and achieve. But as a final thought, imagine the interview as a race, a competitive event where the prize is success. Stress is the large dog that suddenly takes chase, and whilst it's unpleasant to be chased, it does tend to have the effect of making us run faster with determined clarity as we race towards the finishing line. Stress is the dog that chases us, pushing us onwards with determination, forcing us forwards with clarity. Don't be the candidate who buckles under pressure and stress, who gives up and just sits by the side of the track as the other candidates sprint ahead—keep on running.

To deal with stress is to be organized. When pushed to your limits, you need to know exactly what you are doing and why you are doing it in life. This might involve making lists, running your life to agendas and prioritizing those things most important. The stress of an impending interview forces you to be selfish, it pushes you into a position of essential narcissism—this is for the greater good, because it is likely that were you to be successful in the interview those around you would also reap the benefits of your reward. Focus on what you need to, and with some explanation the world around you will understand. Stress is intimately linked to anxiety, and you have possibly identified particularly stressful trigger thoughts or events that make you feel anxious—you should embrace stress in the same way you are trying to embrace anxiety. Stress is your ally in this process, not your enemy. Stress will allow you to run faster, and with the adrenaline from the anxiety you now embrace rather than deny, you will be sprinting as fast as you possibly can.

To utilize stress is to extract its value and apply it even at those times when you don't feel as stressed. This is usually the opposite of what you might do during stressful times, i.e. reducing your stress levels however you can. Here we will embrace stress, and just as we might run faster and more efficiently with the dog in chase, we will also run faster in the same efficient way when the metaphorical dog isn't actually there. During stressful times focus your attention, write lists and agendas, prioritize your time and be determined in your objective. Do this whilst appreciating the fact that at this moment in life, you matter. When you feel less stressed, as you might if you focus and prioritize as suggested, then continue acting in the same way as you did whilst stressed—be essentially narcissistic, and focus your attention to the task at hand.

Reforming, reaffirming, and maintaining

However successful you are in reframing your stress and anxiety into a useful companion on your journey through the interview process, you will often find the unpleasant feelings start to leak out. Stress and anxiety need to be actively and dynamically reformed into a positive force, and just as overwhelming fear of the chasing dog will creep in if you let it, the interview can easily overwhelm you with its critical importance. Actively work on this, using the exercise and words in this chapter if they help, and keep stress and anxiety as useful allies in this process. Hold onto the core principle that these things are useful in the interview process, and instead of stifling them, embrace them into your preparation and interview execution. Actively maintain this position by exercising your ability to sit with anxiety, be mindful, and locate the stress and anxiety in your body, visualize it and examine it as you might an interesting stone on a crowded pebbled beach. In this way, any stress or anxiety in the interview itself will not phase or disadvantage you—indeed, stress and anxiety in the interview will be familiar and welcomed, and will allow you to be the best you can be. You are mindfully present in the moment, both now and during your interview. You are accepting the uncomfortable sensation of muscle pain as you psychologically weight lift because without the pain there would be no growth. The muscle pain tells us we are gaining muscle. The interview pain tells us that we are doing the best that we can.

Further reading

Harding, D. (2014) 'Chapter 4: Reframing anxiety', in *Deconstructing the OSCE*. Oxford University Press, Oxford.

CHAPTER 7

From internal to external

CONTENTS

Operating externally

A key to interview success is the ability to step outside of one's internal world and into the external space around us; to break free of the shackles of rumination and contemplation inside, and to exist wholly in the interview space outside. In the interview we should aspire to operate externally, and whilst we will inevitably need to dip inside to reflect and think about answers to questions, these answers should be moulded and adapted in accordance with the situation that surrounds us. Operating externally also has the advantage of pulling us out of our potential internal fear and paralysis, and allows us to modulate our performance depending on what it actually occurring in the room, rather than being guided just by our internal state. Much of this book is about moving from the internal to the external, and an external objective standpoint will put you in the best possible position for interview success.

Communication: A psychological approach

When we communicate and interface with the world outside, we are forced from our internal shell into the outside world. The interview is important to us, a critical moment in life that can quite literally change the direction of our destiny—because of this, the balance is shifted towards a position where we might prefer to stay inside to make absolutely sure that what we are doing and saying in the interview is exactly right. Whereas we might normally be dragged out into the real world to interact and communicate, when it comes to our interview we might emerge less readily, since the interaction is so much more important than usual and we absolutely need to get this right. This is important. The interview quite literally forces us into a more reflective position in life, and even if we might normally contribute to discussions with little thought or reflection, the interview will force us to be more contemplative in our approach. It always feels impressive when a person actually reflects and thinks before they answer a question, rather than blurting the first thing that comes to mind, and in the interview we must actively reflect and carefully consider our answers before we speak—but instead of dwelling internally, we will reflect in the outside space, amongst the dynamic factors and events that are actually occurring around us. In that way, our answers will be driven not just by what we think is the correct response, but also by the body language and attitude of the interviewer or panel, by our connection with the room and experience itself, as well as all the things we bring into that space with our physical presence.

Communication is our method of interfacing with the world, it is the way we disseminate our internal thoughts, attitudes, beliefs and feelings with the external objects around us. When the communicative stakes are higher, for example, whilst being reprimanded by an angry colleague or confided in by a weeping friend, our communication goes beyond just what we think is the correct response inside—in these high stakes instances we must carefully measure and judge our communication with *theory of mind* (see Chapter 12) and our estimation of the mental state of the other person. We could just reply to the angry colleague defensively, and to the weeping friend logically, but for the best response we should also take their emotional state and wellbeing into account and answer accordingly. We should respond to the encounter and interface as a whole by listening, processing, reflecting, and reacting accordingly. The interview is a high stakes interaction and in it you should apply the same reflective process as you would an angry colleague or weeping friend—you should consider the situation as a whole, reflect on how to approach a response whilst taking into account any measurable factors in the external space, e.g. the mental state of the interviewer, and react accordingly.

The power of the non-verbal

Having just spent the morning interviewing potential medical students, the power and importance of the non-verbal is at the forefront of my mind. Your non-verbal communication with the interviewer is absolutely critical, and whilst it might not change exactly what you say and how they score your answers, it will give an important impression that might be at odds with your excellent answers. So much of our non-verbal communication is driven by unconscious factors beyond our overt control, and it is important to be as mindful of these as possible and to apply all of our communications in the interview thoughtfully and deliberately. As an interview candidate, just as you don't want to appear too nervous by wringing your fingers, you also don't want to appear to over-familiar or confident by leaning forwards and bulldozing through questions with little regard for anything other than yourself. You should tread carefully but not tentatively—like most things, this is a delicate balance. It is important to find a tonic stable mid-point in the interview, where you are sitting comfortably upright with your arms and body relaxed, but not too relaxed. This is your base position, and during the interview it is useful to modify this stance according to requirements. For example, if you need to express vibrancy, confidence, and enthusiasm then it might be appropriate to be more effusive in your body language by smiling and sitting more forwards—but apply such overt confidence with care, and only do so thoughtfully. If you present yourself as too overtly confident from the start then this might appear arrogant or even false. If you are more measured in your approach then applying overt confidence deliberately at an appropriate moment will have real impact, whereas it might be meaningless if you were to be overtly confident throughout. Give yourself the ability to adapt to the interview as required, and do this by starting at a tonic mid-point.

It's important not to over-think things in the interview itself—you need to leave yourself the mental capacity to consider the questions themselves, rather than over-thinking your body language. For that reason, good body language needs to be second nature in the interview, rehearsed, and honed with a cognitive framework of psychological understanding at its backbone. Your body language matters a lot and will tell the interviewer much about your core internal state. Your body language can potentially answer those questions that the interviewer might not give you the chance to verbalize, such as, are you strong enough to cope with this job? Are you sensitive enough to deal with the concerns of our client-base? All of your non-verbal communications will be answering the questions not asked overtly, and you need to be aware of this. Furthermore, your non-verbal communication is a powerful describer of core facets of you as a person, your internal world, and therefore you need to apply any such communications with great care and deliberation. Use hand gestures if it is comfortable, but not too many. The same with facial expressions—use your face to accentuate your opinions and thoughts, but not too much. Apply these things carefully and mindfully. Rehearse your non-verbal communication skills before the interview, and don't waste mental reserves on this in the interview itself. Project your internal world to the external interface with deliberate non-verbal communication, and thereby satisfy your interviewer that you are the right candidate for this position.

Tells and body language

Poker is essentially a game of chance, with a random allocation of dealt cards—what endows a poker player with skill is their ability to control and modulate their body language: their 'tells'. A novice playing poker might be lucky and get a brilliant hand of cards, but they will probably fail by giving their good hand away through body language and tells. A good poker player not only has fine nuanced control of their own body language, telling the world around them only and exactly what they want them to specifically know, but they are also able to read the body language and tells that surround them. Whilst you don't need to be a poker player, and indeed you should operate in the interview with more truth and authenticity than that, you might perhaps embrace the principle and apply some of those skills. At least be aware of them, and aware of what is going on around you. Like all of this, success lies in balance.

It might be that in truth, you really aren't a good fit for this job, and perhaps it is right that your unconscious non-verbal communication and body language should give the interviewer this impression. But it would be a shame for the interviewer to get that impression if it wasn't the case, and unfortunately anxiety and fear can give all the wrong unconscious impressions about you. Being aware of your body language and tells is a good first step, the next is to be gently aware of those of the interviewer though don't dwell upon them. Just apply your body language deliberately and thoughtfully, and be aware of the impression you might inadvertently give if you allow your unconscious tells to reveal themselves. We will think more about body language in Chapter 11.

Disseminating a thought process

Disseminating a thought process, translating an internal process across our interface with the external world, is not as easy as merely stating facts or spouting pre-rehearsed answers. This takes care and skill, and whilst we are all doing this many times every day, doing so in the interview takes particular care and proficiency. When asked a question, particularly a challenging one, we dip into our mind and pull out building blocks of core beliefs, attitudes, and knowledge that are then moulded into a process of thought that has to make sense to the interviewer. This process is the main conduit between our internal world, of which the interviewer wants some insight, and the external space around us. It is not as simple as whether or not you know the answer to a particular question—often the interviewer will want to see your process in action, to see you cope with more difficult questions or problems, and to watch you reason and problem-solve live in the room. As such, just rehearsing answers to questions is not enough—you should also rehearse a strategy in disseminating a logical and emotionally congruent stream of thoughts from your internal world to the external one around you.

We will think later about forming an authentic narrative (Chapter 15) but for now consider the components that make up an answer to a question—this includes a required knowledge of pertinent facts, alongside your underlying beliefs surrounding the question, and any emotional facets from your own experience and understanding of these. A good answer will be based primarily in fact, but will also be coloured by the other more nebulous aspects that lie inside. Some questions may be wholly interested in more nebulous thoughts and beliefs on a topic, especially those that stray into greyer ethical and moral areas—these are essentially guided by your beliefs, experience, and moral code, but the process is the same. Rather than just answering a question, consider how you are constructing that answer, and try to colour your thought process with something that is meaningful to you. Don't always crowbar your beliefs into answers—sometimes, probably most times, you just need to answer questions in a straightforward way. But by being aware of this process, and by rehearsing your skills beforehand, you will be less likely to inadvertently colour your response with more personal and emotive factors that perhaps aren't relevant, or may be misleading.

When disseminating a thought process, after a moment of reflection you should try to apply structure—construct the thoughts around a framework that makes sense. You might want to think about time course or impact, something that has an inbuilt dimensional aspect (i.e. short-term to long-term), or structure around categories that make sense (e.g. local, systemic)—try to hang your thoughts onto a structure the interviewer will immediately recognize and feel comfortable with, then fill in the areas as you see fit. For this to be an adaptive transferrable skill in the interview it really doesn't matter what the question is, indeed the content of your rehearsal questions don't matter—what matters is the way you translate your internal thoughts into the external space, and this method can be applied to any question. There are other aspects of technique that can improve the quality of your dissemination, and these include signposting and the illusion of structure, but we will discuss these in greater depth later in this book (Chapter 11).

CHAPTER 8

Confidence and self-belief

A psychological scaffolding

Confidence and self-belief, in the context of a job interview, is born from our conviction that we are the right person for this job and the knowledge that we've done all we can in preparing for the interview. However, it is likely that we are aspiring towards a new role beyond our current level of responsibility and beyond our comfortable zone of confidence. We are likely to be stretching ourselves farther in life, and as such cannot simply depend on innate confidence and self-belief—here we must carefully construct our confidence upon a psychological scaffolding that takes into account our lack of confidence and experience in this new role. Just being confident is not enough—we must balance our overt confidence with an understanding and appreciation that this new role is a stretch for us, beyond what we are used to and past our comfortable zone of operation. This is true confidence—the authentic confidence that is instilled with an acceptance of doubt. Without some thought applied to this, any doubt at all can crack an external sheet of fragile false confidence, and whilst you may not intend to inject any doubt into your narrative, you cannot control what the interviewer brings to the interaction. It is often the case that an interviewer will deliberately introduce doubt into your narrative, to push you to your limits and check the robustness of your claims of competence. Therefore, our confidence must have doubt inbuilt, as a part of its infrastructure. We must be mindfully confident, whilst also holding onto our lack of confidence and self-doubt—from this is born true confidence and self-belief in the interview.

Of course, not all confidence is based in fact, i.e. based in knowledge and experience of a particular job—many people have boundless confidence whatever the situation, or at least they give that impression to the world around them. Whether this confidence is truthful and authentic is in some ways irrelevant, what matters is that you may be in competition with such a person. It's worth remembering though that too much confidence can be just as off-putting to an interviewer as not enough, and so the candidate who has boundless confidence despite a lack of experience and relevant knowledge is not necessarily at an advantage to you. But if the interviewer is desperate for a safe pair of hands for this particular job, then a candidate's apparent confidence can be very attractive whether or not it's truthful. Also, for many jobs appearance means everything—if you are the kind of candidate who exudes confidence then you are likely also to be confident with the job's client-base, and that in itself can be very attractive, if not essential. Throughout this book you have been building a psychological scaffolding, working on core facets of your psychological makeup to optimize your performance in the interview. Here we will try to bring that together, and will think about how you might improve your own confidence and self-belief in this highly competitive process.

Being robust and resilient

Being robust and resilient is essential in a competitive process such as the interview, especially considering that this is a process that will continue for most of your life. If you are always successful in interviews then you are not afforded the opportunity of building resilience—this only comes from the pain and processing following rejection. Perhaps you might not need to be interview-resilient if you are always successful, but perhaps constant success just reflects the fact that you are not pushing yourself enough in life. Even the most successful people in life face rejection, some face it constantly. Being robust enough to deal with rejection is an essential human quality, and is vital if you are aspiring for a career that takes you beyond the confines of your current situation, if you are reaching higher or further in life. You should be failing, you should be rejected—only with these setbacks can you develop the robustness of character and belief to achieve even greater heights. With this, we should reflect on our past failures and consider their value in getting us to this point in life.

A critical ingredient in the development of resilience after failure and rejection, is the ability to reflect truthfully on what went wrong. If we just attribute the failure to something external, beyond our control, or something unfair and unjust, then we are not allowing ourselves the important opportunity to reflect truly on what went wrong with us, inside. This is a painful process, but an essential one, and we have considered failure earlier in this book (Chapter 4). With truthful reflection we can start to understand our failings, and can work towards making them right. To be truly robust and resilient in the interview process, is to welcome the possibility that you might fail, and to recognize how essential that might be when considering your entire career trajectory.

Things happen for a reason, and whilst it might feel bad to fail, it might turn out to be the best thing that happened in the future. I mention this not to undermine your confidence or to sabotage your chances in the interview, but to encourage you to approach an interview from a position of deference, humility, and personal reflection. There is something very powerful psychologically about already accepting the worst that can happen—it has the effect of making us less worried about a possible disaster, and ironically can make us perform better in a way that makes disaster less likely. It's a bit like trying to fall asleep when you absolutely have to sleep for something important the next day—as soon as you truly accept the fact that you won't sleep all night, you will inevitable drop off. But also, I believe that authentic true confidence and self-belief in the interview is only really possibly when you accept the fact that failure is okay, and that if you were to fail then you would only grow as a person and candidate.

Clothing: A psychological perspective

There are many rules and standards when it comes to your choice of interview attire, and these change depending on the type and seniority of whatever profession you are interviewing for. In general, smart professional attire is required—this is respectful both to the process and the interviewer, and is expected in most situations. Here though we are more interested in what happens psychologically, both for us and the interviewer, and the impact of our attire on how we feel and perform on the day.

Your interview outfit is closely linked to your sense of confidence, and choosing the right clothes can make you feel very confident. However, if you overreach your innate confidence—born from your psychological framework, reflection, and resilience—then you can easily be deflated by the wrong dissecting interview question, and clothing that might have initially made you feel more confident can become a leaden weight dragging you down into the chair. You need to wear clothing that pulls your confidence up slightly, but not too much; attire that is not too far removed from what you would wear day-to-day in this new job and indeed what you wear currently. Balancing comfort with smart professionalism is important, not just because of how you feel but because of how the interviewer feels about you as a candidate. There needs to be congruency between the way you come across, in terms of verbal and non-verbal communication and body language, and how you are dressed. Ideally your attire should pull your confidence levels up slightly, so that you are performing as you might in this new role—from a psychological perspective you are literally stepping into the shoes of a person who will be successful in the interview and right for the job. None of these things are critical, but an appreciation of some of the psychological factors behind your choice of interview attire might be helpful in this process, and could be worth considering.

Throughout this book you will find anecdote boxes with some comments, thoughts and suggestions about the interview process. Anecdotes are a rich source of information about the interview, and you should collect them from bosses, colleagues, and friends whenever you can. Here we reflect on an excellent candidate with an unconventional approach to interview attire (see Box 8.1).

BOX 8.1 **ANECDOTE**

He's a nice chap, but tell him to wear a tie ...

A good friend and colleague had an interview with a person I knew. He performed brilliantly and got the job, but the interviewer had this piece of informal advice.

Reflection: In the case of this candidate, his formidable skills and confidence were such that dressing as he would for work, smartly but with no tie, just about allowed him to get away with this. He felt more authentic and confident with no tie, and feels inauthentic when he dresses smarter than he normally might. In his case, the lack of tie reinforced his warmth, confidence, and abilities—but as a rule always wear a tie, i.e. dress smartly and respectfully, following convention and not standing out from the crowd. This also speaks to our sense of authenticity, and our need to kick any psychological barriers to touch—if we feel inauthentic when we dress smartly like all the other candidates, then this needs to be addressed.

Seeing what they see

I have spoken about shifting perspectives a few times in this book, and have pointed out that such a shift is an important part of being a potentially successful candidate. In this chapter we are interested in developing a true confidence, not a fragile sheet of confidence that can be easily cracked by the interviewer. We want a confidence that is robust and resilient, and to do that we must step outside and see ourselves through the eyes of the interviewer. Here we can be brutal, perhaps not in the interview itself but certainly in the days and weeks preparing for it. Why would the interviewer appoint you to this position? What faults would they see? What are your weaknesses? If you were them, would you appoint yourself? What makes you better than the next candidate? By taking a good hard look at ourselves before the interview, through the eyes of the interviewer, we can be more confident and self-aware in the interview itself. It is rather like having a strong limitations section in the discussion of an academic paper or thesis—a strong appreciation and reflection of weakness actually makes the finished product that much stronger and robust to scrutiny.

Optimization and belief

Only by being truthful with ourselves about our limitations can we find authentic confidence in the interview; only by accepting our weakness can we find true strength. Indeed, denial of weakness will only tend to entrench it. To optimize our performance we need to pull it apart, reflect on all the problems, and rebuild from the ground up. If we do this, then we can start to develop a true sense of belief in our abilities as interview candidates. However, belief in ourselves as interview candidates is very separate from belief in ourselves as people. The interview is just a demonstration of who we are as people, and it needs to incorporate a skillset that is developed, refined, and applied deliberately. This is very different to an innate knowledge and belief that we are good and competent successful people in life. This distinction is important, especially if we fail in the interview—failing in an interview is not failing in life. But whilst different, belief in ourselves as humans is the fire and drive that can elevate our self-belief as candidates, and though not linked, the first can fuel the second.

To be successful in an interview we must surely start with the premise that we are the right person for this job. Whilst I have spoken at length on the value of accepting rejection and starting from a point of humility, embracing the reality of the possibility of failure—at the heart of it, we must assume going into an interview that we are the best candidate for the post. We find this position by travelling through a process of real self-reflection and the acceptance of doubt, but this is all work that happens in the days and weeks before the interview. And whilst we might sit in the interview and accept the fact that we might fail, we must also believe that we will succeed. Achieving self-belief that we will succeed by travelling through the rocky waters of self-doubt and failure will only make our belief that much stronger, that much more robust. Traverse these waters and you will be a stronger candidate.

Being the best we can be

The main objective of this book is to help you be the best you can be. So far we have been pulling ourselves apart in a rather brutal way, exposing our worst parts and losing any defences that might soften the sting of failure and rejection. We have been disregarding those things that make us feel better and less anxious, and instead have embraced anxiety as an essential part of this process. Perhaps you might have expected a different book, one that nurtures your defences and makes you feel better, a book that tells you that failure is not about you being rejected as a person, it is just about that particular interview. You will have realized by now that this is not that kind of book. We have lots of work left to do, and the next two parts of this book are also not designed to make you feel better or more relaxed. In fact, quite the opposite. But our common objective here is to help you achieve your fullest potential in the interview, and I believe that to do that you need to take a long hard look at yourself in the mirror, you need to drop the façade of fragile defence and become a truly authentic and confident candidate. This is possible and eminently achievable, it just takes hard work and a psychological framework of understanding. I hope we have found a way to develop this within part one of the book, and we will build on some of the concepts as we move forwards. Lose your ego and find the real authentic you, the person who can be successful in the interview. Be the best you can be, and reach those heights to which you aspire.

PART 2

A PRAGMATIC
APPROACH

CHAPTER 9

Rehearsal strategies

CONTENTS

Interview rehearsal

Like most challenging tasks in life, rehearsal helps us to improve our performance, and with the interview, rehearsal is essential. We all tend to rehearse interviews naturally anyway, since most of us will have several of them as we progress towards what we hope is the final destination in our career. Rehearsal is an important part of this process, but too much rehearsal can actually put us at a disadvantage and like most things it needs to be done mindfully in the right way, with a sense of balance. Being over-rehearsed will make us feel more confident outside the room, and inside the room might equip us with an arsenal of facts to combat any potential question—but knowing exactly what to say is not necessarily in our favour, and we might miss less overt things at play in the room while we trundle off down our well-rehearsed pathways of fact. It is of course important to have a robust understanding of the facts and figures required for an interview, the content, but don't neglect the other things going on in the room, those other unsaid questions upon which you might be judged just as critically. Being over-rehearsed might make us miss subtleties in questions, it might make us steam onwards when what we should do is spend a moment reflecting and thinking, there and then, about what the right answer is. The answer to a question formulated in the room itself will unconsciously take into account many other things at play in the room, and will be a stronger response because of that—an over-rehearsed response feels safer but totally neglects all the other things happening in the room, including our own mental state. I would suggest rehearsing extensively, with a colleague, group, or friend if possible, but to concentrate on the processes rather than the content. The content can be learnt elsewhere—rehearsal with others is an invaluable opportunity to refine those aspects of your performance that are impossible to work on alone, i.e. the way you come across, and how well you can read the room.

Groups and courses

A clinical director recently told me that he can spot interview candidates who have done lots of interview courses instantly—these candidates tend to fall into set patterns of behaviour, and whilst it might seem to be commendable to have done all that preparation, the interviewer might feel that they are not meeting the actual person. Being too rehearsed, with a clear idea about how these things should be approached can appear inauthentic and disingenuous, and ironically although they may say the right things, the over-rehearsed candidate may be more likely to be disconnected from the external interview experience itself. Being too polished can potentially push you into a more internal position, following patterns and pathways already decided before you even walk into the room, and can take you away from the visceral complex experience in the interview itself. For example, when asked a question about service improvements, a candidate fresh from an interview course might start by saying that there are seven facets to this and reel them off in a structured way— but whilst this is fine from the perspective of interview content, it potentially misses the complex processes at play in the room entirely. The process of the interview is what actually happens in the room: the complex social interfaces and interactions; the non-verbal communications and tells; the empathy—all of these things reach beyond just the content. This book is mainly concerned with the processes at play in the room, for a good reason—whilst the content is important, in some ways the content is entirely expected as a minimum requirement. The way you interact and come across to the interviewer in those more nebulous process-driven ways will be equal in weight if not more important than the content, and in this age of standardized interviews where the questions are often well known a month before the interview, these distinguishing things are even more crucial.

However, that said, interview groups and courses can be extremely helpful and worthwhile if we are aware of the wider processes at play, and are not just approaching the interview like an over-rehearsed automaton. Just rehearsing interview answers in front of others can be very useful in itself, and allowing yourself the vulnerability to formulate and be pushed beyond your limits of comfort in a group can be significantly formative. There are many interview courses available and they are definitely worth trying. It is equally important to rehearse in a less structured way with a group of like-minded individuals, although finding such a group might be difficult. The interview is a competitive process, and however collegiate you may be it might be difficult to find colleagues willing to share and refine their interview skills with a direct competitor. This is perhaps easier if the objective of the group is to refine processes rather than content skills, but still, this is a challenge in a competitive interview process. If you can find willing friends you trust then these are perhaps the best resource for your interview rehearsal. But one of the key roles of this book is to highlight the critical importance of the wider processes at play in the interview, to take the focus away from the content, and in doing so to encourage candidates to form interview rehearsal groups within their professional workplace. I suggest that this is extremely helpful, and will proceed in this chapter with the assumption and hope that this is achievable in your workplace.

One thing to consider, when deciding the membership of your interview rehearsal group, is that this must be a *safe* place. A group is a place to be vulnerable, a place to grow and to be brave enough to say things that are probably wrong. Safety is critical, especially considering the fact that it is likely the other group members are in direct competition with you, if not now then in the future. Such competitiveness tends to draw the worst out of us, and even if not consciously driven, group members might work to undermine each other. This must not be allowed to happen. Group members must be recruited and then asked to move on—this is a no-blame relationship and divorce if needed. If a group member wants to bully and undermine then it really isn't fair on them to be a member of your safe reflective group, they need to join a likeminded group of bullies. To develop during group rehearsal is to become vulnerable, and with this you can develop a trusting way of gently feeding back and nurturing each other's skills and attributes. If the group is well balanced and safe then this is an excellent melting pot of differing strengths and allowed weaknesses—allowing weakness is critical, and with some group reflection all can become stronger.

A rehearsal group can also be a useful way of collating information about a particular workplace, although this would require dealing with the unfortunate fact that several group members may be in direct competition for a particular position. In medicine and surgery, it is likely that candidates will be applying to a particular Trust with several positions available, or perhaps different positions within the same institution. Whatever the process, either within the group or individually, it is important to research your potential workplace. Not doing so will probably be immediately obvious to the interviewer (see Box 9.1).

BOX 9.1 ANECDOTE

Such as shame they didn't know a thing about us ...

A colleague's genuine disappointment that a candidate had not researched the unit they had applied to work in at all, and knew nothing about what made this particular unit special.

Reflection: Research is essential before your interview—you need to know enough about the workplace to justify and explain your reasons for wanting to work there, but also need to know what makes that particular place unique and special. For the staff, what makes them feel proud to work there? Knowledge of this is essential. In this anecdote my colleague was genuinely disappointed for the candidate as they seemed very nice, but was also rather offended that they had no knowledge of the unit. It seemed totally remiss of them to not have shown any curiosity in the unit, and appeared to demonstrate a pattern of working and a lack of inquiry that was unattractive and not right for the unit. Consider the impact that your lack of inquiry and research might have on the interviewer, and the conclusions they may draw from this potentially innocent oversight.

Modelling and feedback

As a general group rehearsal strategy, I suggest that rather than being intent on covering as many questions as possible, concentrate on a specific question or task in a session and model this amongst the group. By modelling I mean to repeat the question, around the group in turn, with each taking the role of interviewer and candidate sequentially while the other members observe and take notes. It is a way for the group to model and refine an approach to an answer, and to optimize that process rather than just covering more required facts and content. When the question is run over a few minutes each time, observers should make note of non-technical skills, empathy, and body language instead of just the content—content is important, but is so often the focus at the expense of other process skills. Concentrate on the process skills and refine these within the group as the question rotates around the table.

Regarding feedback, this should be done with care. Try to separate facts from feelings, i.e. first discuss the facts of the rehearsal, how the ideal scenario would run, and then discuss the feelings, how it made you feel. Try not to contaminate the facts with your feelings, and vice versa. Give the interviewee the opportunity to feedback first, so they can address anything that could have been better before being told the same by someone else, and always try to use constructive feedback. There is no room for ruthless criticism or judgement here, the interview rehearsal group is a safe space where all should grow—but if something about a performance can be improved then find a respectful way of saying that. Honesty is important, but take care not to inadvertently undermine one another's confidence.

Applied empathy

We have previously considered empathy in some detail (Chapter 5) and have discussed its value as both a disseminator and detector of subtle verbal and non-verbal communications. Empathy is an important part of your rehearsal, and each group member should make efforts to apply this innate human quality as an applied skill. Be an empathic candidate in the way you connect with the interviewer, and try to put yourself into their mind, see yourself through their eyes. Aim for a human connection during rehearsal, something that feels important and authentic, a connection that has emotional weight. Think of empathy as a skill you can apply between one and ten, as though you have a control slider you can increase if you'd like to ratchet up the emotional interpersonal connection and understanding. This is your *empathy tone*—apply more tone and you will be more overtly connected with the interaction. You should definitely not just rehearse the required content mechanically with no thought or emotion—indeed, to do so is just a waste. In your rehearsal group you have a fantastic opportunity to practice and hone your empathy, and in doing so you will optimize your ability to communicate and collaborate with the interviewer.

In the next exercise we will consider a strategy for interview group rehearsal (Exercise 9.1).

EXERCISE 9.1 A PANORAMIC PERSEPECTIVE

In your interview rehearsal group, assign tasks to all members and take it in turns to rotate a scenario or question around the table. The interviewer and interviewee rotate, unless you have a senior mentor or colleague offering to interview in which case they retain the interviewer role. The others in the group observe and make notes on what was said, how the interviewee came across and the non-verbal communications that occurred—these should be divided up so that one observer is, for example, wholly noting the non-verbal. Choose a relatively open question or scenario that is wide and generic but relevant for your particular upcoming interview. For example, describe what makes you the right candidate for this job, rather than a specific closed technical question with a very specific required response. Give yourselves two minutes on a timer, ask the question as it might be said in the interview, and give the interviewee the time and space to answer in the best way they can.

Once the question is over, spend a few minutes feeding back before rotating to the next person. In the feedback think about the whole performance with a panoramic perspective, but allow the interviewee to do this first. Try to make a comment about the following facets of the scenario: the content in terms of quality, depth, and breadth; the fluency of speech; the non-verbal communications and body language; the empathy; the atmosphere during the interaction; the eye contact; and any other facets of the interaction that arose. Don't just focus on the literal content—the depth and breadth is more important than what was actually said, and the myriad of other factors present during the interaction must not be neglected. Once the interviewee has been through these facets from their perspective, the other members and interviewer should feed back in a similar way, keeping the feedback constructive and positive, and avoiding judgement and criticism. Don't tell the interviewee how they could have done things better, instead try to show them that when the interview scenario rotates around to you.

Video feedback

Video is a harsh, unforgiving critic, and watching back an interview rehearsal can be agonizing. But this is an extremely useful way of getting a totally objective perspective and set of eyes, and can be especially useful when combined with group feedback as described earlier in 'Modelling and feedback'. Spend time picking apart a performance, watch and discuss, and get as much value as you can from the encounter. Notice as much as you can—the real value is in the detail, and don't let any small detail slide. Video is also useful when rehearsing alone, and whilst the camera itself can change the way you perform, this is probably not that different from your performance being modified by the presence of others in the actual interview room itself. Video can feel very exposing but no more so than the interview itself, and getting used to this level of exposure is a good thing. Make yourself as vulnerable as possible during interview rehearsal, expose every weakness and flaw, and thereby build up true strength and resilience for the interview itself.

CHAPTER 10

A psychological arsenal

CONTENTS

Psychological optimization

The first step in optimizing our psychological makeup is in understanding and accepting that this is a journey that will take our entire lives—whilst we can aspire to be psychologically optimized, we will probably never fully achieve that. However, we can strive to be as psychologically mindful and enlightened as possible, and such a mind state is very helpful in the processes surrounding the interview. Sometimes in life, the realization that something isn't perfect and could be better is in itself powerful in affecting growth and change. As an analogy, a brilliant singer will always aspire to improve, with an acute knowledge and understanding of their current vocal flaws—indeed, this understanding of what isn't right is the very thing that pushes them towards vocal mastery and brilliance. A mediocre or bad singer, by contrast, will be happy just to sing in the shower and think they are great. An acceptance of weakness is essential for true strength, and an appreciation of our lack of mastery is essential in achieving mastery. For the interview, to be the best you can be, it is helpful to be psychological mindful and connected to the experience, and whilst this might be a level of mastery we might never fully achieve, the importance lies in our journey towards mastery rather than the final acquisition of this. It would be extremely helpful in the interview to be in possession of a framework of psychological understanding, and the first part of this book worked towards that aim. A framework of psychological understanding allows us to check in and reality check throughout the interview, to be more mindful of the psychological factors at play in the room, and to be more aware of our own mental state—it will improve our ability to perform well in the interview, and is an essential weapon in our arsenal of interview skills.

Reality checking

Reality checking is the process of checking in with yourself and your environment as you go about the business of living, and doing so can give you useful information about why you might feel a particular way. For example, if you are feeling stressed and overwhelmed with a headache, it could be a natural assumption that the headache results from the stress, and perhaps it does. But checking in allows you to apply a psychological process around this, and you might realize that you are thirsty, having not drunk enough fluid, which is then impacting on your mental and physical wellbeing and causing the headache. Reality checking is taking a moment to STOP and reflect on how you are feeling in this actual moment, in this actual room, rather than being awash with over-riding and overwhelming emotions. If you feel paralysed with fear or anxiety in the interview STOP, reflect on the chair you are sitting on, the air you are breathing, and think for a moment about your emotional state. Take a sip of water, gather yourself, and carry on. Reality checking is also helpful if the interview feels as though it is lost to you, out of control—this might have arisen from your reeling after a disastrous question or task, or you may just feel overwhelmed by the experience itself. Stop. Think about the room, the noises the temperature, the noises outside the window, the crooked tie of the interviewer—give yourself a moment to reflect on this reality that you occupy here and now, and focus on one small detail of it. Distract yourself by thinking, just for a moment, about the interviewer tying his tie as he looked into the mirror this morning, or the bird that's just about audible outside the window. These tangible facts ground you into reality and allow you to grapple back into the present. Then you can carry on with the interview. Rehearse reality checking in the days and weeks leading up to the interview, and arm yourself with this useful psychological skill.

Calmness in chaos

Whatever happens in the interview, you are the calm eye at the centre of the storm. Indeed, whatever chaos you find yourself surrounded by in life, you are situated in the calm and will only be pulled into the whirlwind if you step away from this calm, centred spot. Imagine a movie from the perspective of the protagonist in a plane crash: the image slows as the person breathes and remembers their life up to this point—chaos only exists if we allow it. Whatever happens, we can breathe and centre ourselves, ground ourselves in the moment, and achieve a state of internal calm. With this calm we can spend a moment to reflect and properly think about whatever task may befall us, be it a question or challenging moment in the interview. Sometimes it is useful to have a way of distracting yourself back into your centre of calm, and whilst snapping an elastic band on your wrist might not work in the interview itself it could certainly work in the moments just before, outside the interview room. Find a way of psychologically snapping yourself out of the chaos around you, and ground yourself, here and now, sitting here in the room. Practise this during chaotic moments in life, for example, being crammed into a claustrophobic tube carriage with people arguing and coughing all around—instead of listening to music, just centre yourself and relax, be aware of the chaos around you, and reflect on your centred position of calm. Focus on the calm and ground your thoughts into this moment. Rehearse this and employ it if you need to in the interview.

Being mindful

We have discussed being mindful several times already in this book, and I hope you agree that being mindfully connected to the actual moment during an interview is a worthwhile psychological state to aspire to. Mindfulness is our ability to exist purely in the moment and focus all of our resources to the task at hand; it is understanding the context of that task whilst having an appreciation of what is going through the minds of others in the room—whether or not you actually know what they are thinking, the important thing is that you are aware they are thinking something. A good exercise for achieving a state of mindfulness uses a photograph: find a photograph from the internet that speaks to you, be it a countryside vista or a painting of the sea. Print a copy of the photograph and carry it with you. When you are next in a coffee shop or on the tube, take out the picture and look at it. Spend three or four minutes just looking at the picture and thinking about what you can see there, what is actually going on in the scene. Focus on the photograph, and whilst you remain aware of what is going on around you, empty that from your mind and just think about the small details in the picture. Construct a narrative within the picture, i.e. imagine who took it or painted it, imagine what circumstances led to them capturing this scene, then think about how it might be relevant to you. If you get distracted by a noise in the external world, perhaps a person who just bumped into you, then pay attention to that and allow it into your mind, but then accept the distraction as part of the moment, here and now, and immerse yourself back into the picture. A person bumping into you is not your focus, but the fact that it happened is important and is part of this present experience, here and now. Accept the distractions with gratitude and know that they have contributed to the moment that you are currently experiencing, and once accepted assimilate them and go back to your task of immersing yourself in the colours and brush strokes. With practice this will allow you to achieve a more mindful state of being, one that incorporates the external distractions without letting them pull you away from the centering task at hand. You will then be able to do this in your interview, and will be more successful as a result of it.

Operating externally

With every interaction between now and your interview, operate externally. Do this by stepping outside of your internal world and considering any interactions from the perspective of an external observer. During a conversation don't think about what you wish to say next, instead focus entirely on what the other person is telling you. Don't think about how their words make you feel or what you will be doing next, instead really think about what they are saying and consider what drives them to say these things. Project yourself into their minds, as best you can, and see the interaction from their perspective. Next, think about the environment, their body language, the objects around, and the noises just beyond sight. Embrace the external world and position yourself amongst it, look at yourself from out there and don't allow yourself the indulgence of operating internally. Operating externally during your interview will improve your performance, so learn to do this as best you can before then.

Focus on the task at hand. This might appear to be an obvious statement, but after internally formulating your own goals and objectives in response to a particular task or interview question, focus on achieving this goal externally within the context of whatever is happening in the room. The goal or objective is formulated internally, but needs to be achieved externally in the world around you, rather than held and dealt with internally. Ensure that the interviewer can see exactly where you are going with a particular task or question, read the room around you, and moderate your journey accordingly. The analogy would be a maths question in an examination—the examiner needs to see your workings and thought processes clearly written down, and sometimes these rough notes will be just as important as the final answer. Be transparent in your thinking and signpost your thought processes if needed—this is better than trying to work all of this out internally and just presenting the interviewer with the answer you think they are looking for. They are probably just as interested in the journey as they are the destination. Do this with focus (see Box 10.1).

Identification

Consider some of the unconscious psychological processes that are occurring within you and within those around us. These are the things that drive our behaviours and are often born from childhood or traumatic experiences. One concept is identification, and if you have suffered a childhood trauma then you might be holding different psychological identifications inside, for example, the abused and the abuser. It is often the case that an abused person will identify with

BOX 10.1 **ANECDOTE**

He was all over the place. How could we trust he would change if he worked here?

This is a description of a candidate who lacked focus in the interview.

Reflection: Focus in the interview is important and you should follow threads of thought through to their conclusion, but this has to be balanced with breadth of knowledge and ensuring that all the bases are covered. In this case the interviewer got the impression that the candidate lacked focus, so whatever the candidate's strategy was, it failed. The impression of the interviewer is critical and we must employ skills in reading their non-verbal communication and body language to get a register of this. Whilst I wasn't in that interview, I imagine that the interviewer's exasperation at the candidate's lack of focus was palpable in the room. Also, the interview is in essence a mutual collaboration, and the candidate probably felt that frustration on some level if the interviewer experienced it so strongly. Consider the feelings in the room—if the room feels chaotic to you then it probably feels that way to the interviewer too. Be guided by the abstract sense of atmosphere in the room, and if something is going wrong, try to fix it.

the abuser rather than the abused, since identifying with the abused is just too painful. Therapy can sometimes unlock this and allow an abused person to identify with, and eventually embrace, the abused position, allowing them to finally pay attention to and find compassion for the abused person within them. This ultimately leads to peace and recovery. Whilst I don't want to make light of this important psychological process, it did occur to me writing this book that perhaps it might be useful to think about identification in the context of the interview. Some candidates walk in with boundless confidence—they undoubtedly identify with a person who is successful and gets the job. Another person is less confident, and perhaps they have been more worn down by previous failed interviews and therefore identify with a person who fails and doesn't get the job. We can't just change who or what we unconsciously identify with, but sometimes just being aware of a potential unconscious psychological process provides enough in sight and understanding to overcome such base identifications. Don't be over-confident or under-confident—consider what position you might be identifying with, and don't let your subconscious put you at a selective disadvantage. Perhaps choose to dis-identify from these things—and although such a choice could be considered futile against the powerful tide of the unconscious being, choosing to dis-identify might be a helpful position to foster in the interview. In fact you are choosing a conscious locus of control, and whilst it might not be fully successful in stifling the subconscious elements that drive all of our behaviours in life, at least you are making an active choice.

Being bulletproof

Of course, no one is bulletproof, and even as an analogy for resilience it doesn't really work—but it is a good state to consciously aspire to. Bullets hurt, and our unrealistic fantasy of bullets painlessly bouncing off us will never happen. However, we can move towards a state of being bulletproof if we can merely survive the painful bullets, and with time be able to function even whilst being shot. Rather than building psychological defences that make bullets bounce off us causing no pain, we should aspire to developing the kind of skin that can still be shot at but retains the ability to process the pain and move on. When something happens that causes pain in the interview itself or the days and weeks preceding, don't deny that pain pretending it doesn't hurt. It hurts. It would hurt anyone to be shot in this way. Instead, register the pain, process it, and understand it within your wider framework of psychological understanding, then move on. This is being bulletproof.

CHAPTER 11

Communication skills

CONTENTS

A psychological context

Communication is the way we disseminate our internal world and thought processes out into the external space, the way that we connect with those around us. The accuracy of our dissemination is critical if we are to properly and satisfactorily communicate our internal world, but our accuracy can be impacted upon significantly when we are under pressure and duress. For sound accuracy we need to be centred, calm, grounded in the moment, and be able to express our thoughts and feelings carefully. In this way, all of our psychological framework and skills are essential components in delivering an accurate representation of our internal space to the world around us. In this chapter we will think about some skills and techniques that might help us feel calm and centred, and will help us to disseminate accurately to the interviewer.

Verbal communication

Whilst your attention and focus will be directed on what you actually say in the interview, you are communicating much more to the interviewer than just the overt verbal, but this is a good starting point to consider. The content required for any particular question in your particular field is beyond the remit of this book, it should be known and be second nature. Here we are concerned with refining our interview process skills and being the best we can be. It is worth considering that even in standardized medical and surgical interviews where the questions are pre-published for candidates and therefore the content delivered to the interviewer will be very similar, the way that content is delivered differs significantly from one interviewee to the next. This is partly down to innate communication skills and fluency, but perhaps also the differing underlying beliefs and ideologies between candidates that drive the overtly similar content. It is these differences that make some candidates score higher than others, as such underlying ideologies give the interviewer a sense and insight into you as a person and doctor, and what you might bring to this particular job and career pathway. So whilst both the candidate and interviewer might be frustratingly constrained by a standardized pre-published script, many things can be verbally communicated and heard beyond the boundaries of the required standardized content. It is worth bearing this in mind—be aware of your own underlying beliefs and ideologies, and how these might influence your verbal communication during the interview.

Any verbal communication during your interview should aim to be fluent, concise, inclusive, and as short as possible, lasting no more than a couple of minutes. Don't fill time with rambling content—keep answers short and succinct whilst addressing the core question asked. Before even speaking, ensure that you fully understand exactly what is being asked of you and spend a moment reflecting before answering. Every word you deliver should be thoughtfully considered and ultimately relevant. The tone of your speech should be measured and constant, as should the volume and rate. Just speak normally and as warmly as you can, given the circumstances, but whilst retaining a sense of professionalism and authority. You need to be confident but not too confident—this is a balance. Try to avoid vocal 'tics', such as repeatedly saying 'you know', or using the word 'absolutely' too much. Incidentally, rarely is anything in life absolute, especially in health care. Avoid too many 'um' or 'ah' noises, although some vocal tics will be unavoidable since you will have been employing them for a lifetime. Just try to communicate your thoughts as accurately and concisely as possible, and string words together in a fluent and understandable way. We will spend time on developing an authentic narrative later in this book (see Chapter 15).

A colleague recently told me that his problem in interviews lies in his humility and reluctance to speak highly of himself. Speaking highly of himself by saying that he is the best person for this job, or even good enough for this job, feels wrong and boastful, it feels inauthentic to him. He struggles in speaking positively about himself and instead falls back to an authentic position of humility and self-deprecation. Whilst this position is perhaps quintessentially British, such attitudes and approaches have no place in the interview and need to be kicked to touch as soon as possible. If this is the case for you, then you simply need to practise talking about yourself in a more positive way, ideally with colleagues, with content that reflects fact and authenticity. Your verbal communication must lead the way in this task, and in time your non-verbal expressions will follow.

Depth and breadth

Regarding the content you deliver in the interview, a consideration of depth and breadth is critical in pitching your answer correctly regardless of the subject matter. Some answers will require just a short answer, but many questions will have greater depths you could delve into and wider edges towards which you could stray—you need to find the limits of the answer yourself, and doing that requires an understanding of what the interviewer might expect along with being able to read the room and pick up on any available cues and clues. A useful approach is to cover the content concisely but to hint at a wider understanding of the issues, in terms of depth and breadth, to the interviewer. You could overtly offer to speak in more detail should they wish, or just drop in some pertinent facts that could lead them down a rabbit hole should they choose to follow. Regarding breadth, it's usually good to indicate briefly that you understand the more widespread implications about whatever you are speaking of, and especially if these implications breach other disciplines or professional realms. An appreciation of how your particular area fits into the wider context is always useful, and it is good to give an indication to the interviewer that you understand this and are happy to speak about it if they wish. However, keep these added insights in terms of depth and breadth very much in your back pocket, and do not play all your cards unless there is a specific reason or request to do so. Be concise but do so with the mutual understanding that you could speak further on this subject if needed but are choosing not to right now.

Non-verbal communication and expression

An awareness of our non-verbal communication and expression in the interview is crucial for success. Often these will act as 'tells', informing the interviewer about our innermost neuroses and workings, answering questions not even asked—but with due thought and attention they can be tamed and used to our advantage. Our non-verbal communication, without further processing and modulation, will tend to reflect our core emotional state and underlying belief structure. If we are anxious, worried about failure, and of the belief that we will fail, then this will be communicated loud and clear to the interviewer via the non-verbal. Likewise, if we feel that the position is in some way beneath us, we might appear flippant and disrespectful. Sometimes our non-verbal communications will reflect a particular defence, for example, if we are terrified of failure and surround ourselves with a fragile defensive shield of confidence then we might appear over-confident, but are likely to also appear inauthentic. It is almost impossible to hide our underlying core state from the interviewer, and if we exert effort in trying to do so we are diverting energy away from the important task at hand. Our non-verbal communication and expression needs to reflect a candidate who is confident but not too confident, who wants this job and who truly believes that they are the right person for it—the best way of achieving this is to make it so. If your core underlying state is a problem, then you need to address these issues and build your confidence from the ground up. However, there are some ways that we can modulate our non-verbal communication and expression, and we will consider these next.

Body language and facial expression

From the moment you walk into your interview, and indeed for the weeks and months of preparation leading up to that point, you need to be in control of your body language and facial expressions. This basic skill is absolutely essential and relatively easy to master. Perhaps an important start in this is the realization and acceptance of the impact that these non-verbal communications can have on the interviewer. They reflect your internal world and can give away aspects of your anxiety and neuroses that simply should not be present during the interview. More so, if you can tame these unconscious aspects of your communication to the interviewer then you can use them to your advantage, and give a better impression of yourself that is positive and affirming. The way to tame your body language is to use body language as an overt skill in the interview, in the same way a poker player uses their tells to manipulate the other players (see Chapter 5). Body language is your demonstration of empathy, the way you can non-verbally connect with the interviewer, and to neglect this core skill in the interview is to put yourself instantly at a disadvantage to others employing the skill.

When you walk into your interview change the position of the chair slightly before you sit. Move the glass of water in front of you so it is comfortably within reach, then smile and make eye contact with the interviewer or panel. It will feel alien to smile in such a stressful and important interaction, you might literally feel your cheeks fight back against the shape, but smile you must. Once you have smiled once, politely and professionally, then you can smile again if needed but might not wish to. It is in your control, and you have set a threshold—rather like testing the limit of a reclining chair before sitting down. You should set your body language and facial expression at a tonic mid-point, sitting upright but not too straight, your face warm but not too warm, your arms relaxed and hands comfortable in your lap or resting on the table. Make eye contact with the interviewer or the panel members in turn, and maintain a natural eye contact throughout. Don't stare at your hands or at the wall, you need to maintain eye contact. If this is uncomfortable then focus on the point between the eyebrows—this gives the impression of good eye contact and actually feels less intense for the other person. Pitch your tonic mid-point as you might sit on the front row of a lecture, respectful of the speaker and curious as to what they might say. Be curious about your interviewer, imagine what they are thinking and feeling—this is your starting point. Also take in the room and ground yourself in the present moment, as we have discussed earlier in this book (see Chapter 3, Exercise 3.1).

When you move a part of your body, such as moving your hands in an expressive way or taking a sip of water, do so deliberately. Every movement will be registered by the interviewer, and although they may not make any assumption at all from whatever you do, it is helpful for you to be mindful of their constant observation. You should not feel self-conscious or worried about moving, indeed you should not be dwelling inside your head at all—as we have discussed extensively, you should be occupying the external space and be existing well outside the self-indulgent realms of narcissism and introspection. We simply do not have the time for an indulgence of introspection at this point, and we need to operate externally. If you move your body you do so purposefully and consciously, and in doing so you will be pulling yourself out of any potential introspective ruminations and back into the external space. Operate externally. Every movement contributes to what is happening in this room, in this very moment, and every movement is critical and within your locus of control.

Use your body language and facial expression to complement and contribute to whatever you might wish to verbally communicate to the interviewer. It you feel passionately enthusiastic about something don't place the weight of this wholly in your verbal communication—instead, keep your voice steady and controlled, and express the enthusiasm with a subtle change in facial expression and subtly increased hand movements. Note the word subtle—overly employed body and facial expressions must be dialled down, and only subtle movements in combination with congruent verbal communication will do here. Any movement, facial expression, or noise that is too extreme or dramatic will be off-putting—you must be measured and controlled at all times. Your body language and facial expression are conduits for your expression of empathy, and through these let the interviewer know that you can connect in a sophisticated social way, both with them and with the general public if you were to get the job. If something is said that makes you feel sad, or you get the sense that it might be appropriate to express sadness, then you might drop your shoulders and head slightly alongside a subtle frown. If you feel happy you might express this with your body and face, but again, in a subtle measured way. I recently had a potential medical student confidently leaning forwards in his chair and even winking at one point—don't do that. You should at all times be the consummate professional with a strong physical identification that mirrors your suitability of this post—not too confident but not too humble. It's a balance, and a tightrope you need to walk throughout this whole process. Just be aware that you are walking a tightrope and this will all fall into place naturally. Don't blunder out without even realizing a balance has to be struck, as you will quickly stumble and fall.

Words have weight

Words, and indeed pauses, have weight. We have spent much of this book considering the unspoken words in this process, but it is also worth reflecting on the fact that every word spoken is important. Choose words wisely, and before blurting them out, spend a moment to reflect. Doing well in an interview is not about choosing complex words, it is often about stripping back to the simplest possible word. This is because we are not trying to join a self-congratulatory club that excludes others; we are aspiring towards a job that interfaces with the world around us, and it is important to be able to communicate with as many people in that world as possible. Also, it is much more impressive to be able to express a complex idea in simple terms, and therefore using the simplest possible words will give you immediate plaudits. Be concise and precise, and use the simplest words to convey your thoughts and ideas to the interviewer and world around you. If you use a word that gives the wrong impression, and you realize that in the interview, you should correct it. Don't leave it hanging there—just apologize and use the correct word. The wrong words have weight too, and will often drift around the interview room long after you have left it. Think about the words you decide to employ, and use them carefully and deliberately.

Consider also the amount of words you use. Try to develop the ever-elusive skill of concisely capturing a train of thought, employing brevity whenever possible, but don't waste too much energy on this. It's inevitable that sometimes you will say too much; sometimes you will need to be more verbose to communicate a complex thought process, but aim for brevity rather than complexity. In a pragmatic sense, just don't say too much. Keep sentences short, and keep answers concise and to the point. Make the interviewer's job easy, not hard, and let them move through their required questions as seamlessly as possible (see Box 11.1).

BOX 11.1 ANECDOTE

Just too much speaking, it was impossible to get anywhere ...

There is only so much time for an interview, time is a rigid boundary that will not shift. Speaking too much reduces the potential to be asked more questions.

Reflection: It is difficult to be concise and brief, especially when we are trying to express something that might be complicated, or trying to convince others of our worth. Being concise and brief is essential for the interview, but not too brief—the question needs to be answered, but always assume you are doing so against the clock. Your speech should not be rushed or garbled, indeed it should be calm and measured with pauses as needed, but should be as succinct as possible. The interviewer should not feel frustrated that they can't move you on. Try to read the interviewer and get a sense from them whether you are speaking too much or too little, but as a default be succinct rather than overly verbose.

Signposting and summarizing

When you communicate, do so in a way that is easily digested and understood by the interviewer. It is critical that the interviewer hears and registers the points you are making, and for success it is important to facilitate this as best you can. Rather than speaking in a block of text, punctuate your speech with headings and sub-headings. Do this overtly and deliberately. Tell the interviewer exactly what you are going to talk about it, then do so, but do so in a structured way. We will think more about forming a narrative thread to your speech later in this book (see Chapter 15) but for now just consider the importance of applying a common-sense framework to whatever you are communicating. This should be a framework that is possibly familiar to the interviewer, but certainly one that makes sense to them. Punctuate the speech with key points in the frame, so that the headings make a coherent whole that makes sense overall.

I have already suggested that you need to be concise and succinct in your answers, but if you get the impression that the interviewer hasn't really got the point you wanted to make, or perhaps you haven't made it as well as you could have, summarizing is a useful skill. Good summarizing in an interview is extremely difficult to do and would certainly require proper rehearsal, especially considering the time constraints and constant pressure from the interviewer to move on.

However, if you really do wish to reiterate a train of thought then you can succinctly round up the points in the form of a bullet-pointed list. This might appear too rehearsed or clumsy and I wouldn't recommend that you summarize routinely in the interview, but you can if you absolutely must, and to do so is better than an important point being missed by the interviewer.

The illusion of structure

When you formulate an answer to a question live in the interview, the thoughts will inevitably be a jumbled mass, mixed in with underlying beliefs, ideologies, and emotions. Without further processing this would emerge, at best, as a block of text, and if truly formulated live then there simply might not be time to signpost, i.e. to add in the headings and sub-headings. We only have so much capacity and if a question is unexpected and particularly oblique or challenging, it will be enough to be able to give any cogent response at all. But here, rather than speaking in a block of inaccessible text, you should apply the *illusion of structure*. Add in slight pauses, arrange and assign headings as you go, and give the illusion to the interviewer that your thoughts do indeed have structure. In some ways, you should always be adding the illusion of structure to all your speech. Even with headings and sub-headings in place, adrenaline will tend to push you on and make you speak at a faster rate than normal—slow yourself down, add slight pauses, and reflect on the words live as you speak them. This gives the illusion of control. Indeed, this is control.

Let us now work on improving the quality of our dissemination, accuracy, and fluency of newly formulated speech—the next exercise will help with that (Exercise 11.1).

> ### EXERCISE 11.1 DISSEMINATION, ACCURACY, AND FLUENCY
>
> In this exercise we will use video or audio recordings to capture our speech, ideally video so that non-verbal communications and expressions are also stored. Set up the camera so it will capture your entire upper body and position a laptop or tablet computer in front of you. Search the internet for 'oil painting urban landscape', select the images, and click on the first image. Set a timer for two minutes, and then speak about the picture. Describe the content as accurately and concisely as possible, using the simplest possible words, and also employ body language and facial expression to the task. Don't stare wholly at the picture, glance down periodically but hold your gaze into the lens of the camera. Be as fluent as possible, and aim for a flow of melodic-sounding speech that is easy to listen to. Verbal fluency is absolutely critical in the interview and this is the place to refine that. When the timer goes off, stop and watch this back. Then, choose the next picture, set the timer, and repeat. Rehearse this exercise daily until you can accurately disseminate your thoughts regarding the pictures. Use other search terms if you prefer.

Learning to listen

Listening is a process beyond just hearing sound, it is about registering all of the verbal and non-verbal communications directed at you in the interview. Doing so properly in the interview takes care and attention, and must be a process that is actively pursued at all times. Every communication is potentially important and you cannot miss any of them. You should actively listen, and be seen to do so. Pay attention to every word spoken, and ask the interviewer to repeat a question if you don't fully understand it. Pay attention also to the interviewer's body language and facial expression, as well as the feeling you experience when they speak to you. Your own feelings, in response to the interviewer, are useful sources of information in your overall reading of the interview room.

To do this efficiently in the interview you should overtly rehearse this outside the room, in the days and weeks before. Listen to the world around you and register every communication directed at you, beyond just the verbal. Try not to miss anything, and get into the habit of doing this routinely. Good, effective communication is very much a two-way-street, and receiving information is just as critical as disseminating it.

The expert communicator

A true expert in communication would know that they still have much to learn, and that mastery will probably be ever elusive. We can all learn more, and communication, our link to the world around us, will probably take a lifetime to master. However skilled we can always improve—indeed, the realization that things can be better is often what makes a communicator skilled in the first place. It is all about refining and improving, and this is a gradual process that should be in balance with the need to authentically and honestly just say whatever you think and feel in the interview. If you feel paralysed with anxiety then perhaps that is important, and it might tell you that this isn't the right pathway for you in life. But more often than not, your emotional state in this highly pressured and crucial psychological encounter might deceive you, and tell you you can't do it when you can. You don't need to be an expert communicator, you just need to be the best you can be and not let underlying neuroses and anxieties drag you back. Also, realizing that the best communicators are also self-critical about their performance should hopefully give you some comfort in knowing that you are not alone in this. The very best communicators are constantly learning and improving—you should join them.

CHAPTER 12

Situational awareness

CONTENTS

Theory of mind

Theory of mind is the ability to put yourself into the mind of the interviewer and see the interaction from their perspective. It is your ability to mentalize,[1] to see the world through their eyes, and to be guided by what you imagine to be their motivations and expectations. Some psychiatric illnesses, such as autism spectrum disorder, reduce a person's ability to conceptualize what others might be thinking, and others, such as paranoid schizophrenia, give a person an inflated impression of their knowledge of what others think. The stress and pressure of an interview can push us from a stable position of mental good health towards one or other extreme, and we might find ourselves less able to conceptualize the thinking of the interviewer when faced with the overwhelming task of the interview itself. Having a robust theory of mind is not essential for success in the interview, but it is useful to have a working understanding of what the interviewer might be thinking and expecting. It also has the advantage of pulling us from our internal space, forcing us out of the shadows of neuroses and rumination and into the light of the interview room outside.

Motive and motivations

When you walk into your interview, immediately put yourself into the mind of the interviewer. See the scene through their eyes, and as you ground yourself and connect with the moment in the room think about your silhouette from their perspective as you take your seat. You are filling a shape previously filled by another candidate, you are repeating a task just completed by another—you are one of a list, and the anonymity of that harsh truth should be reassuring. You must also ensure that through the eyes of the interviewer you will stand out from the crowd, but not because of who you are—it is because of what you say here and now, and how you react to this encounter. Your motive is to make the interviewer notice you for all the right reasons, and for them to realize that you are the ideal person for this job.

As the interview progresses and you are asked a string a questions, keep checking in on what you conceptualize to be the driving motivations of the interviewer in this encounter. Where are they going with this thread, and what do they want from you? Think beyond the literal—what is driving their enquiry? Are they anxious about your ability to deliver in this position? If so, how can you allay their anxiety? Look below the surface and consider what drives the interviewer with every question. When a question is asked and you take a moment to reflect, incorporate your conceptualization of the driving motivations of the interviewer into your thoughts and reflections on this actual question. It might be apparent from the string of questions that the interviewer is trying to establish the potential for you being a trusted pair of hands if you were to get this job, and if so that might colour your answers accordingly. Or you might get the sense the interviewer is concerned about whether or not you are capable of this amount of responsibility, and in that case you might add that consideration into your reflection and answer formulation. At the very least, checking in with your conceptualization of the interviewer's motivations will pull you out of your own head and into the external space, and will also act to debunk and demystify any perceptions or fears you may have of the interviewer. In truth we can never really understand what actually drives the interviewer, but by applying ourselves to the conceptualization of this we are effectively pulling ourselves towards the very real interface between us.

Filling the required space

As your silhouette takes a seat in the interview, from the perspective of the interviewer, consider for a moment the potential space in this room. The interview is structured around empty space, designed wholly for you to occupy. There are set questions and the interviewer takes their seat in the room, but the other empty chair and the empty space between the asked questions is there for you to fill. You fill this space with your physical presence and your communications, both verbal and non-verbal, and whilst this all might seem perfectly obvious I think it is useful to be minded of this space. Instead of just speaking when there is a gap, consciously and overtly fill the space provided for you in the room with your voice and body language. Don't overfill the space, i.e. don't speak too loudly or for too long, don't have overly expressive hand gestures and be a dominating presence in the room—just slot into the space provided, and fill it with a similar amount of volume and movement already provided by the interviewer. In this way, match the volume of your voice and the degree of body movement roughly to that of the interviewer, and seamlessly fill the space left for you, not more and not less. If you over-fill the space with too much volume and over-enthusiastic manic energy then you will appear overbearing to the interviewer; if you under-fill the space by speaking quietly and being completely still and timid then you will appear to be lacklustre and lacking in confidence. If you choose to speak quietly, particularly at a certain point in the interview, then that is fine—but be mindful of the space to fill, and accentuate your quiet tone with subtle facial expression and hand movements. The combination of speech and movement adds together to fill the space, and you need to moderate both to ensure you don't over-fill. You should certainly never be speaking loudly and using wildly expressive hand gestures—if you need to raise your voice then you should be entirely still. This is just a different psychological way of approaching the interview space, to help you fit seamlessly into the pre-existing tone in the room, and to further pull you out of the indulgent and damaging recesses of your internal introspective world. Operate externally, in this space.

Being curious

Curiosity is an interesting state of being, and tends to have the psychological effect of pulling us out of primal emotional states in any given stressful situation. When training as a medical student I was extremely squeamish during operations, but this reduced as soon as I found my sense of curiosity towards the process. If you feel scared in a situation, you will find that being curious about your surroundings will partly allay your fear. Curiosity empowers us psychologically by changing the dynamic in a given situation, since instead of just been a passive player in a scene we are now an investigator. It gives us a sense of control and allows us to view a scenario from a slightly different perspective. It is useful to approach the interview with a sense of curiosity, and when you walk into the interview room be curious about the space and its occupants—nurture your flame of curiosity as the interaction progresses. It is extremely flattering if a person shows genuine curiosity in you, and the interviewer will likewise be flattered. Adopting a curious standpoint also has the advantage of pulling you out of yourself and into the room around you, and as you can see, we are working hard in this chapter to find different and novel psychological ways of doing just that.

The following exercise will help you ground yourself into the interview space, and remain grounded even when the waters become more rocky and turbulent (Exercise 12.1).

EXERCISE 12.1 FINDING YOUR ANCHOR

This exercise is an extension of Exercise 3.1: Reading the room (Chapter 3), and by now you should be familiar with the concept of reading the room. As we previously discussed, think of the interview space being made up of concrete objects, material elements, and abstract qualities. To remind you, concrete objects are the chair, table, interviewer, and lamp—those concrete things around you in the room. Your physical presence in the chair is also a concrete object adding to the dynamic of the interview room. Material elements are the air you breathe, the dust that falls through a sliver of sunlight hanging in the air, the noise of a drainpipe just outside the window, and the sound of the interviewer—the material elements are the working currency in the room, the oil that makes the machine work. These are not the only things here in the room, there are also the abstract qualities: the atmosphere, the sense of tension or claustrophobia, perhaps a sense of space and exposure. The abstract qualities perfuse the material and concrete elements, infusing them with meaning. You are already armed with this psychological framework of understanding, and when you occupy the interview space with your physical presence you can anchor yourself into the present moment by utilizing this framework.

When you walk into the interview room, and once you are settled in your chair, focus your attention for a moment on something in the room, either concrete, material or abstract, whatever brings itself immediately to your attention. It might be the cup of water in front of you on the table. The cup might be plastic or ceramic. This is the concrete element. The water might be so cold that condensation has formed around the plastic base. Perhaps there is a small puddle of water around the base—the material. The cup was placed there to ensure that you are adequately hydrated, but more than that, it is there to ensure that you are comfortable. It demonstrates the interviewers care for you as a human being. Care—the abstract. Noticing all this is instantaneous, but it has a powerful psychological effect—it grounds you in the room, in this very moment. The plastic cup is an anchor point, tethering you mindfully into the present, holding you here safely while you operate externally and apply yourself to the task at hand. If during the interview you find yourself retreating back inside your own mind, find another concrete element in the room, whatever grabs your attention first, and use this to pull yourself back into the room. Reflect for a moment on the material and abstract, and anchor yourself in the room. Perhaps the slightly open window, or the interviewer's crooked tie. Use these things to anchor yourself mindfully into the moment, into the external space of the interview room, and start again to operate externally. If you find yourself drifting away into internal rumination and introspection, look out into the external space and find an anchor. Tether yourself externally, and exist out here in the light.

Understanding the interviewer

If you get the opportunity to be an interviewer yourself, take it, as this is the best way to understand the processes essential for this role. Being the interviewer during rehearsal is a good second-best, but will not give you an experience of the necessary detachment required for good interviewing. Whilst this role is largely about being human and finding a candidate who will fit into the workplace, you need to appreciate that there are several candidates in competition and the more human and caring the interviewer is, the more diligent they will be in terms of being fair and transparent. It is difficult not to get drawn in and either care, or care less, for the interviewee—but to be a good objective interviewer a degree of objective, dispassionate, detachment is required. The interviewer is being wholly professional, and if they appear dispassionate and uncaring then that perhaps reflects the fact that they actually care a lot. Of course, there may be occasions when an interviewer prefers a candidate that they already know, and since there is little we can do about this it isn't worth concerning ourselves with. What we can be concerned with is the fact that the interviewer wants to care more about one particular candidate, and that they will feel more satisfied giving the job to a person they have a good feeling about who also ticks all the required boxes, rather than a person they don't warm to but fulfils the necessary criteria. It might be that the best candidate on paper and in the room is not the person the interviewer warmed to most, and inevitably this person might get chosen. But do not underestimate the unsaid questions in the room, and consider the fact that we all want to work with people we get on well with.

The interviewer will usually start from a detached, professional, and objective starting point, and as the candidate it is your job to use empathy skills to draw them away from their detached place into the warm interface between you both. We are all human, and however detached we try to be, we can all be drawn to a warmer, more human place. This is especially the case given that the interviewer is probably personally invested in this appointment, and choosing the right person will probably significantly impact on their own working life. Use your empathy and non-verbal communication skills to show the interviewer that you are human, that you would be a great person to work with, and that you would love this job. This is of course a balance, and one to be added in moderation with your professional presentation of your skills and attributes. But add a sprinkling of humanity in there too. Perhaps it might be appropriate to apply some humour, but do so with extreme care—it is a wonderful plus to get a genuine chuckle from the interviewer, but this will be very rare. The best you can hope for is in drawing them away from their detached objective and standardized position of fairness and equality, and letting them see the good person you are beyond all that formality. To try to understand the interviewer will add to your situational awareness, but as we discussed earlier, we can never really know what drives them. We can, however, aspire to know that—and your curiosity regarding their drivers and motivations in itself can place you in a stronger and more enlightened psychological position.

If you have ever experienced being an interviewer yourself, and have interviewed a string of candidates already shortlisted and thereby fulfilling the minimum criteria for appointment, you will know that whilst you are of course looking for attributes that make a particular candidate stand out from the crowd in a positive way, you are also highly attuned to any factors that make a candidate unsuitable. As an interview candidate, once you are past the shortlisting phase, the old adage 'the job is yours to lose' really is relevant. Honesty and authenticity are critical in an interview, and perhaps it is the case that aspects of your authentic self do make you unsuitable for this post, but try not to give the interviewer any reason to mark you down. One way this might happen is by appearing overly divisive or collusive. There are always two sides to any story, and as a professional potential employee it is important to always try to see both sides, even if it is very obvious to you that one side might be better. If something has gone wrong in a previous job, try to see the situation from both perspectives, rather than encouraging the interviewer to collude with your own perspective. The interviewer is a human being, and as humans we are naturally drawn towards empathy and collusion; but as an interviewer they must remain objective and see both sides. Be aware of this potential conflict in your interview, and try not to draw the interviewer away from their comfortable neutral position by pulling them towards your own view when discussing previous difficulties (see Box 12.1).

I wonder what they would say about me ...

About a candidate who criticized a previous employer in their interview.

Reflection: As a candidate do not criticize previous employers or colleagues in the interview, even if you feel genuinely aggrieved. It just looks bad, and reflects badly on both your professional discretion and character. Try to be benevolent and be reflective if you have to mention any prior grievances, and overtly contemplate the situation from the perspective of the other person. There are always two sides to a story, and with this situation you need to be able to reflect on both—in this way a prior grievance can actually work in your favour, as it can show the interviewer that you were able to reflect and rise above such challenging situations.

Reference

1. Bateman, A. and Fonagy, P. (2013) Mentalization-based treatment. *Psychoanal Inq*, **33**(**6**): 595–613.

CHAPTER 13

Reviewing and refining

CONTENTS

Practice and processes

The interview is a critical event that can have significant repercussions for our future livelihoods and wellbeing; it is a charged psychological encounter with great weight and meaning, and we need to approach it with the respect it deserves. This book has so far strived to equip you with a psychological framework of understanding, a new novel psychological standpoint from which to tackle this hurdle afresh, and has also tried to suggest some pragmatic approaches to help achieve this. A common message so far has been to accept weakness and anxiety, and through vulnerability to find true and authentic strength. Another guiding principle is the idea that mastery is only possible if one is open and accepting of our infinite lack of mastery, i.e. that this is an aspiration we may never actually reach. Realizing our fallibility gives us the psychological footing to climb higher and achieve more—if we were to feel infallible we would be satisfied and would climb no higher.

This idea is relevant here, and whilst you have been equipped with a psychological arsenal for your interview, to maintain and develop this takes practice and nurturing. Go through the chapters in this book and refine your core psychological state and skillset, work on your attributes and weaknesses from the ground up. Concentrate on interview processes rather than content—the specific content required for this particular interview is of course essential, but the processes are relevant for every single interview you will ever do. With every next interview, whether a failure or success, you will gather and refine your interview process skills—and with a framework of psychological understanding underpinning your progress you will stack up your new and refined skills in a way that makes sense.

A passive skillset

The processes we have been considering in this book should form a passive skillset that underpins and drives your performance in the interview, rather than being active skills that need to be consciously considered and employed. I have mentioned several times when a skill should be actively applied, such as empathy and listening skills, but even these need to drift back into a passive set of behaviours that are very much second nature and natural to you in the interview. This will occur with practice and rehearsal. The interview is a challenging task and you need to be able to commit all your cognitive and emotional resources to the task; you should not be spending efforts on finding an anchor or trying to empathically connect—these things should be passive and second nature. There is clearly a conflict here, and I have suggested many things so far that should be applied, yet now I am saying they should drift back to the passive position. Consider a child learning to walk, having to concentrate on every step at first but in time being able to walk whilst performing other more complex tasks—yet the walking still takes some thought. It is a passive innate skill, but requires constant monitoring and refinement—your psychological skillset is rather like this.

Being present is the key

I won't repeat myself yet again, and those of you who have read to here will have heard me make this point many times throughout the text. Just be present. Cooking a meal is a good example of us being present in the moment, being connected to the sights and smells as we concentrate on the task, carefully chopping so as to avoid injury, watching the meal develop in front of us as we facilitate the process step-by-step. Writing and performing music is much the same, as are many tasks that require focus and concentration for their success. It is so easy to dwell introspectively during an interview, to be burdened by what you should or shouldn't say, to be shackled by past failures or rivals you perceive to be better—this is not good, and is simply not helpful in the interview. If you were to paint a landscape from the confines of your own neuroses and mind, you would inevitably miss the finer details that might have otherwise brought the painting to life. We should probably aspire to be truly present for every moment of our all-too-short lives, and perhaps this is something you already do—but I hope I have provided a new set of eyes with which to view the interview, and a new position for you to try out next time. Be mindful, both of your own state and the state of the world around you, and give yourself the best springboard for success.

Being an actor

This might appear to be a strange heading given the amount of time and effort we have dedicated to finding our authentic selves so far in this text, but I think that it is an important one. Much of life is acting, and a doctor is as aware of this as anyone. If we were to operate truly authentically as a doctor, truly empathizing and connecting with every patient's pain and distress, then we would surely burn out quickly. We need to find a way of relating to patients in a meaningful way that protects us and preserves our own health and wellbeing. We also need to find the stamina to do more. We do this by acting, though we may not see it as such. We might follow an illness narrative, we might interact in well-formed patterns of behaviour, we might connect in a way that maintains our boundaries yet still feels authentic to the patient—this is essentially acting. Indeed, for talented actors, the process of acting can feel very real indeed, and when we connect with a powerful performance we only believe in it because the actors believe in the role themselves wholeheartedly. They inhabit the role. In some ways, acting is an even more nuanced way of interacting socially, and whilst we are not all great actors, being comfortable with the notion that we can infuse our authentic performance in the interview with a sprinkling of acting is very useful.

The trick to acting in the interview is to realize that the role you are playing is yourself—your ideal self, free from interview neuroses and anxiety, unburdened by past failures, and identifying with a candidate who is successful rather than one who fails. This book so far has been your instruction manual, your set of guidelines to help you inhabit the role of yourself, allowing you to observe your performance as a whole from a more external standpoint and to modify your behaviour as you progress forwards in the interaction. You are not reacting with natural instinctive empathy as you would to a friend over coffee—you are reacting in a purposeful and applied way, as you might if you were acting a scene about a friend over coffee giving you bad news. This is a subtle difference but an important one—for if you accept the premise that the complex psychological factors at play in the interview should be deconstructed and applied deliberately and mindfully, then you are essentially agreeing that you need to authentically act.

Perhaps the truth lies somewhere in between, and I am aware that many candidates are extremely uncomfortable with the idea of acting. Indeed, we have worked very hard so far to step away from the theatre of an inauthentic false interview performance, and moved towards a more genuine and meaningful place of honesty. I just add this section to provoke thought, to add to your arsenal if you so wish, and to perhaps level the playing field slightly with the morass of other less authentic candidates who will act shamelessly. Try stepping into the role of yourself and see how it fits. It might not help, but it might ironically enable you to truly and finally be yourself in the interview.

Whether you are comfortable with being an actor or not, it's important to ensure that the role you inhabit, i.e. your authentic self, is present at any pre-interview event or gathering. Whilst informal events before the interview can be a less pressured way of getting to know your potential place of work, and them getting to know you, you must always operate exactly as you would in the interview. Be authentic at all times, even if this feels like pretence or acting. In truth, if you 'act out' the role of your authentic self, and purposively operate to the best of your capacity, you will probably be more authentic and true to yourself than if you just wander around as yourself, anxious, and defenceless. Shield up. This is a balance (see Box 13.1).

BOX 13.1 ANECDOTE

Don't forget the importance of any pre-interview events such as an informal cheese and wine night the evening before, an informal chat, or visit to the unit ...

This advice was given to me as I was writing this book.

Reflection: Consider what informal pre-interview events and meetings represent for both you and the interviewer—this is a time when soft skills can be gently demonstrated and assessed, and the interviewer can see you as a person before the structured standardized and detached process of the interview itself. This is an important opportunity for you to connect with the interviewer on a more human level, but although it is less formal you should treat it with as much respect and deference as you would the interview itself. Be yourself, but be yourself the professional candidate, rather than yourself the person who likes to drink and sing karaoke.

An intricate construction

The psychological framework of understanding we have been carefully constructing over the preceding chapters is intricate and complex, too intricate to be able to pick apart in the interview when you need to focus all your reserves on the difficult task at hand. Change in life is not easy, and whilst I am not so arrogant as to suggest that a book like this would offer any real change at all, I do think that for change to be possible we must take the time to unpick things from a psychological perspective and rebuild from the ground up. Here we have tried to do that together. It is rather like the Eiffel Tower—layers and layers of thought, planning, and construction resulting in a majestic monument, each step critical for the whole but most of the steps totally inaccessible to those who view it from the outside. What matters is the construction itself, how it looks and feels, and how it functions in the real world. Some of these steps will have more weight for you, some will be meaningless and cast aside, but I hope that you are now in a stronger more mindful psychological position than you were before reading this book. If so, then this is very helpful, as the interview is competitive and closely matched—any edge can make all the difference. Nurture your psychological construction as whole, and test its functionality in interview rehearsal. If you need to work on specific steps then do so, but the important thing is the construction as a whole. Don't get bogged down in details or intricacy, just take on board what resonates and use any of the techniques that present themselves in the interview if you so wish. At the very least, you will have a greater understanding about the psychological makeup of this extremely charged psychological encounter, and perhaps with that knowledge you will learn more from the interaction for next time.

PART 3

GENERIC SKILLS AND STRATEGIES

CHAPTER 14

Skills toolkit 1: Building your toolkit

CONTENTS

What is a skills toolkit?

This book is concerned with psychological underpinnings and interview process skills, and has overtly neglected the consideration of any content that may be required for your specific interview. This was necessary, since this text is designed for any interview regardless of profession, specialty or level, but also I think that stepping outside of the content is useful when approaching interview preparation. We tend to get so hung up on the required content, this will inevitably be the focus in our minds in the days and weeks leading up to the interview, and perhaps rightly so. You will need to find the required content for your specific interview elsewhere, in books or online. But whilst we are not concerned with content in this book, I do think that it is possible to process and store the content required for your specific interview in a way that is both transferrable and easily accessible, and we do this by the employment of a skills toolkit.

A skills toolkit is a psychological receptacle for your collected interview skills—it is a method of categorizing and cataloguing the skills in a way that makes them adaptable and modular, and thereby renders them easily accessible to you in a variety of different tasks and questions. We will start to build a rudimentary toolkit here, and whilst this is perhaps best suited for generic interview skills, specific content skills can also be filed in this way. Rather than entering your interview with learned answers to questions that might or might not come up, or with a script prepared for a pre-published question, instead walk in with your hands free and unburdened, and then deftly reach into your toolkit and retrieve a specific skill should you need it. In this way, you can afford yourself the cognitive space to be able to connect with and read the room, to centre and ground yourself in the moment, and to be guided by all those other nebulous abstract qualities and non-verbal communications present in the room, rather than being full to capacity with prepared and learnt rote answers. In this final part of the book we will then go on to think about some generic skills that might aid you regardless of your profession or specialty, but for now we will start to build our skills toolkit.

From contextual to modular

Content skills, i.e. skills specific for your interview incorporating content and facts that will be required for your interview, are acquired within a particular context. They may be experientially learnt, this is perhaps the best way, or might have been gathered from books or online. They might have been directly taught or developed in your rehearsal group. Wherever and however they were acquired, they were assimilated within a particular context, perhaps with the sole purpose of answering a specific question in your interview. The objective here, in building your skills toolkit, is to convert that contextually acquired skill into a modular form that is adaptable for many different interview scenarios and hurdles, rather than it just being immediately relevant in its original context. This is done by dissecting into the specific contextual skill, considering it as a collection of micro-skills and abilities, and extracting the generic interweaving threads that imbue it with power and utility. Rather than rehearsing and filing the specific contextual skill, we rehearse the extracted generic elements in a variety of different scenarios and situations, and file the skill in this modular adaptable form.

This concept is best explained by an example. Common questions in the interview might ask you to list examples that demonstrate either leadership or initiative—two separate questions with very different answers, and both employing skills and attributes acquired in specific contexts. Whilst these answers are different and should be presented as such, they both contain generic threads and attributes that give them power and utility, and it is these interweaving threads that we wish to extract. If we can mine into these examples and extract generic skills and attributes, then these can be moulded and modulated for use in either question, or both if needed. The other advantage of this dissecting process is that it encourages us to reflect on our skills and attributes, and to understand what it is about these that might be desirable to the interviewer. Then, with this information, we can highlight the facets to give the best impression, and if we are short on time we can do so as concisely as possible. In this way, our skills toolkit will be packed full of high-value generic skills and attributes, all ready for integration and concise dissemination as part of our formulated interview answers.

The following exercise suggests a method for transforming context-specific skills into modular threads that imbue your skills with value (Exercise 14.1 and Figure 14.1).

EXERCISE 14.1 CONSTRUCTING MODULAR THREADS

Consider your model answer to a particular interview question—this could be something very specific or as in the worked example here something more generic, such as giving an example of a time you demonstrated leadership. Take a sheet of A4 paper, divide it into three sections with two horizontal lines, and write the question at the top of the page (see Figure 14.1). Under this, write your model answer as concisely as possible, using a bulleted list if needed—don't fill the page with a long rambling answer, keep the words succinct and to the point, using no more than the upper section of the page. In your answer capture something that means something to you, something that has emotional weight. Under this, divide the middle section of the page into three columns. Label the first column 'thoughts', the second column 'feelings', and the third 'facts'.

Consider the example you describe and recall exactly what happened on the day. Think about the thoughts that went through your head at the time, and also those in your mind right now with this reflection—list the thoughts in the first column. The thoughts capture your thinking at that time and upon reflection—these might be influenced by your core beliefs and ideology, and if so circle these in red. Consider the facts of that specific example, i.e. when, where, who, and how. What were the concrete implications of what happened? The second column grounds the example in context, and with which you could potentially embellish the answer with detail should you wish to form a lengthier narrative. Finally, think about how you felt during the example and list those. Your feelings are an emotional time-stamp, a way for you to travel back there and re-experience the encounter as it happened. They are also

(continued)

EXERCISE 14.1 **(CONTINUED)**

a powerful way for you to disseminate the encounter with meaning and emotional weight to the interviewer.

Whatever your answer, no matter how technical and specific, you should be able to dissect into it and extract relevant thoughts, feelings, and facts. By breaking your answer down into these building blocks you are mining into some of the core psychological skills and attributes that give it power.

Label the lower section of the page 'modular threads'. Here we will list threads of thought, feeling, and fact that interweave through the answer above—these are our modular skills, extracted from the example and stripped away from any specific context. We find these by examining the middle section of the page and finding links between the words written in the three columns. Look for a thought that links to a specific feeling, and find the fact that is most appropriately attributed to both. In the example of leadership, a thought might be something like 'strength', the feeling might be 'compassion', and the fact might be 'grieving'. So in an example that demonstrates your leadership, when you stepped in to lead the team after your boss was unexpectedly taken away from work after the sudden death of a relative, you have extracted: strength; compassion; and grieving. Circle these words in black pen and draw lines between them, linking them together. These are the building blocks of your modular thread—now construct a piece of narrative that combines all three, and captures a core facet of you as a person that contributed to the success of this example. For example, you might write something like: 'In the face of grief I found the strength to be compassionate'.

This is a modular thread, capturing a facet of your character that contributed significantly to the example above, but a facet that could easily be used in other questions and scenarios. This is you as a person, a core attribute, and although you can follow the thread and building blocks back to the point of inception, the thread will stand alone within a different context or example. List other modular threads if you can. These are your modular skills, to be filed into your skills toolkit. List them if that's helpful, or find a way to mentally package them away. Consider them as a collection of modular threads, and extract them for use if needed in the interview.

A modular skillset

The modular threads you have created in Exercise 14.1 are not just generic attributes that could be applied to anyone—they are specific to you. They each contain thought, feeling and fact, and as such have internal context and emotional weight. They mean something, and can be used when the situation warrants it. You have probably always walked into interviews with a sense of your strengths and attributes—this is the same, perhaps just more refined and sophisticated. The difficulty with a nebulous concept of one's excellence is in its delivery—it can tend to sound too generic, and that's if you can overcome your self-deprecation and humility to deliver anything at all. Delving into actual contextual examples and extracting modular threads allows you to speak confidently to your strengths in the interview, and gives you the ability to elaborate with specific hard facts and context should you need to.

Application

In a charged psychological encounter such as the interview, when you need to function at the limits of your cognitive ability, it is sensible to give yourself as much space to manoeuvre as possible. Being armed with a skills toolkit allows your hands to be free and unburdened—rather than being

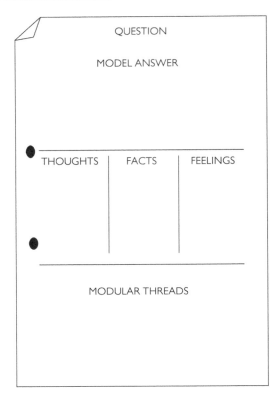

Figure 14.1 Constructing modular threads
Transform context-specific skills into modular threads that imbue your skills with value.

pre-loaded with answers, anecdotes, and examples of personal excellence. If you need any of these things just dip into your toolkit and retrieve a modular skill as required. If you are too burdened with information at the start of the interview, then you will find it that much harder to both connect with the experience and also to choose exactly what you need for any specific question. Instead of carrying these things in with you, enter the room calm, collected, and unburdened. Carrying specific answers to questions reduces your anxiety, so without these rehearsed answers you might feel more anxious—but perhaps that is right. Artificially reducing anxiety by over-rehearsing set answers is unhelpful, and if you need to return to normal undefended levels of anxiety then so be it—better that than being overly defended. You know you have access to modular skills should you need them, and this will act to reassure you. With your hands empty you can properly ground yourself and connect with the room and experience, just as we have been discussing in this book. Then, if you need to, dip into the toolkit, retrieve a modular skill and apply as needed.

In the following skills toolkit chapters we will consider and discuss some further aspects of the interview from a generic and process driven psychological perspective, that might usefully contribute further to your skillset.

Skills toolkit 2: An authentic narrative

The value of narrative

Narrative is story, a thread of commonality that runs through a collection of words and facts, joining them together in a way that makes coherent sense to the listener. Narrative brings us together, both the storyteller and the story-told, joining as we meander our way down through the pathways and passages that link words together. Narrative structure has a start, middle, and end—it follows convention and applies a familiar structure to what might otherwise be just a random collection of facts and events. We all love stories, we are just hard-wired in that way—we are drawn into the narrative, the warm familiar structure pulls us in, we become fascinated by the collection of words and facts because we know there will be a pay-off at the end. We expect it. Narrative has great power, and in this chapter we will consider ways of using narrative to structure our answers in the interview, to draw the interviewer in and pique their genuine curiosity, to render them essentially human within this detached and standardized process.

Being authentic

Consider your interview an opportunity for you to showcase your very own autobiography. While fictional stories can willingly suspend disbelief, the autobiography needs to be grounded in truth and authenticity in order for it to have any power or impact. If we knew that an autobiography was a fiction then there would simply be no point in reading it, despite its plethora of clever narrative tricks designed to draw us into the pages. This is important because a lack of authenticity, from the perspective of the story-told, is not necessarily based on a careful assessment of the known facts, indeed the actual facts can be inconsequential—a lack of authenticity is often perceived because of the way that something is disseminated. As a listener we have keen instincts as to the authenticity and veracity of the teller, and will spot a liar very quickly—this might be because they pause slightly at just the wrong point, because they look away and avoid eye contact from time to time, or perhaps their affect and confidence simply isn't congruent and consistent with what they are actually saying. These things undermine a narrative, even if it was the case that the narrative is totally true and authentic. So for us, as orators in the interview, we need to ensure that our storytelling is not only truly authentic, but that it also appears to be authentic to the listener. We will consider these things here.

Being authentic is having the conviction to stand up for what we believe in, and the ability to back up the claims we make. It is something beyond just truth, it is the encapsulation of truth in the things we say and the way we say them. As a writer of crime fiction and a person who has extensive first-hand experience with serial killers, I was surprised to be told by an assistant agent that my fictional serial killer lacked authenticity. How could they possibly know that? Regardless of my real-world experience, if my narrative does not appear authentic to the listener or reader, then it lacks authenticity. The customer is always right. This might seem unfair but in fact it is absolutely right—we are a social species and the only thing keeping us together is our ability to connect, empathize, and communicate. Starting from a position of truth is only the starting point. Our communication thereafter must be authentic, and for that it needs to comply with certain rules and thresholds that appear congruent with that underlying truth.

Congruence is an important concept and observation in psychiatry, and it refers specifically to the matching up of a person's behaviour and appearance with what they are actually saying. A tearful person who says they feel fantastic appears incongruent, and as a psychiatrist this is concerning. A person who is tearful and says they feel bad appears congruent, and whilst we might then be more or less concerned about the actual mood state, the congruency is reassuring as it implies a degree of authenticity in the person. A person can be authentically incongruent, as they might have a bipolar affective illness with a labile mood that renders them tearful when they genuinely feel great, but this is the exception rather than the rule. The general rule would be to look for congruency between speech and appearance, and this is a rule you should aspire to in the interview. There are subtleties within this rule, and thresholds of incongruence that are tolerable. For example, if you are upset and tearful but putting a 'brave face on it', and are saying you will fight on despite the difficulties, this is incongruous, but it may be tolerable if the emotional weight in the delivery gives the speech enough empathic impact to push it above the threshold required for authenticity. In this case, with good empathy a degree of incongruence can be accepted and still be perceived as authentic, but again, this is not the general rule and although it could happen in an interview, it probably shouldn't.

Aim for congruence between what you say and the way you are coming across to the interviewer. If you say you are excited about this new position then smile and appear so, if you say you are concerned about the safety of infrastructure then look concerned as you say that. This appears straightforward and obvious, but the problem with the high-pressure stakes of an interview is that we invest all of our energy into what we say, and our non-technical softer skills, such as smiling and maintaining eye contact, tend to drop off. Non-technical skills are absolutely critical in the interview and we have a whole chapter dedicated to just this (see Chapter 17), but for now be aware that your presence in the room needs to mirror what you are actually saying.

Eye contact is essential in appearing authentic, and again we will speak about this in more detail later (Chapter 17), but for now always try to maintain a degree of non-threatening eye contact that does not invade the interviewer's personal space. A lack of eye contact is a bad sign for the interviewer, and eye contact is often listed specifically on interview-marking sheets as something they are looking for and marking explicitly. We all know that a lack of eye contact in the interview probably just reflects a lack of confidence, or nervousness, or simply a loss of soft skills as we focus entirely on the required content—but even with this shared understanding, a lack of eye contact is a cardinal sign in the interview, and if you don't have eye contact you will definitely lose marks. In this way, eye contact is merely a hoop that we must all jump through, it is a game that we must all play—including the poor and exhausted interviewer who might have absolutely no appetite for making eye contact with yet another candidate just before lunch. Eye contact will be essential for your interactions with the world at large if you should get this job, so it makes sense that good eye contact in the interview is an absolute requirement. As well as this though, eye contact is a powerful marker of authenticity, and a lack of it gives the strong impression that you are inauthentic.

When considering your perceived authenticity also think about your verbal fluency. Verbal fluency, like eye contact, is often called out specifically on interview marking schemes, and like eye contact is a skill that is obviously important if you were to get the job. Fluency is also a soft, non-technical skill that can fall away under pressure and we have considered it earlier (see Chapter 11), but for now consider how much verbal fluency actually communicates to the interviewer in the room. It communicates intelligence, aptitude, enthusiasm, confidence—the list goes on. It doesn't directly communicate authenticity, but a lack of fluency can give the impression of a lack of authenticity. If you pause and stumble over words when you are telling the interviewer how enthusiastic you feel this will appear inauthentic, and even if the interviewer understands that you are nervous, this lack of authenticity might override any interviewer-compassion resulting from your obvious nervousness. This is because emotions like enthusiasm are primal and instinctive, and should normally stifle any superficial nervousness simply because of their core belief and intensity. Just be aware of this and practice your verbal fluency within the context of this psychological understanding—Exercise 11.1 in Chapter 11 is useful for this purpose.

Finding vulnerability

A critical, key aspect to finding narrative in your answer lies in finding your vulnerability. In movie terms, a script needs a heart. Imagine a movie camera zooming into a close and exposing image of you, then pulling back to a wider shot that includes first the people around you, then the structures surrounding the people. When you answer a question, you should at times try to make yourself vulnerable, by metaphorically pulling the camera in close—by using 'I' statements, and considering how the question relates to you personally. For example, in a question about leadership, you could start your answer by considering what aspects of you, your skills, and personality, make you a good leader. Don't make yourself too vulnerable though, this is a balance. Then, pull back slightly to a wider view, and consider the dynamics of the relationships around you— how do your interpersonal dynamics make you a good leader? Perhaps give a brief example. Finally pull back to a wider shot and consider the question from a systemic perspective—how do your leadership qualities steer and affect your team or service as a whole? Finding your vulnerability and using close-up 'I' statements will draw the listener in and allow them to connect with your narrative, just like in a novel or movie. Then, lead them through your answer as the movie camera pulls back through wider perspectives, through inter-personal, and systemic aspects. This is an aspect to finding your narrative, and of itself can be a useful way of approaching and structuring some interview questions.

A narrative framework

What makes a good story? And in the interview, why would we bother? When asked to speak about your previous career, achievements, and journey up to the point of this job interview, or asked to talk about what makes you the right person for this job, you could neglect anything I might have to say about story and narrative and just blurt out a jumble of unrelated facts and events. You could do that. Or instead, you could structure you answer in a way that will make sense to the interviewer even if they have absolutely no knowledge of the events you describe; instead you could structure in a way that draws the interviewer in and makes them want to know more, even eager to know more. Or you could forget all that and just concentrate on the hard facts, it's really up to you. I suggest that instead of just launching into a regaling of facts and events you take a moment to structure your reply, and consider employing a narrative framework upon which you can attach your facts and events, thereby developing a narrative flow that will in essence be a better self-contained answer to the question.

So back to our initial question—what makes a good story? A story has a beginning, a middle, and an end. These are the first scaffolds you use to construct your narrative framework—a starting point, a journey, and a destination. This is easy when asked to describe your journey up to the point of the interview, the trick is in choosing the right place to start, and pitching the right level of detail for the journey itself. It is the same with a story, movie, or novel—the starting point is critical, as is the level of detail in the journey. Just like a novel, your starting point needs to be a place that is relevant to the interview, but also at the time of a significant event that led to change, ultimately leading on to the journey up to this point. It might be that you were working in an office and had an inspiring encounter that led you to the realization that you needed to get the training and experience that led you to this point. Regarding the journey, don't get bogged down in the details—instead, focus on the emotional journey rather than the practical one, and pepper your emotional process with discrete and interesting facts along the way. So with your training, you found the process enriching and rewarding, particularly the time you ran a team when your boss was away from work. Like all responses, keep it succinct and to the point, completed within a couple of minutes and delivered with conviction and fluency. But frame your experience within the confines of this most basic narrative structure: the beginning, the middle, and the end.

The beginning, middle, and end narrative structure will work for most questions directed at you in the interview, even if the questions don't relate specifically to an overt journey. Whatever they are asking, they are asking for your take on this. The question is ultimately about you as a candidate, whatever they ask, even when they are asking for a list of technical details—it is what you think about, and how you present the list of technical details that is important. The interview is about you, not the facts. Since whatever you say is your own opinion, you can always frame this within a basic narrative arc that starts where your opinion started on this matter, and has a journey up to the present. Your opinion might have evolved, and if so concentrate on the emotional factors that drove this rather than the technical facts—what was is about you, as a person, that made this process evolve, and how did that make you feel? Ground your answer in your humanity, and try to structure it as a personal narrative rather than just a collection of technical facts. Even if they are explicitly asking for the facts, it is you as a human being that they are interested in—the question is merely a vehicle for them to use for that aim. Never forget your story, don't neglect your humanity.

The next component of your narrative framework is the concept of personal conflict leading to resolution. All good stories begin with conflict, and this conflict is resolved as the story reaches its conclusion. Your narrative is exactly the same. What was the trigger that led you to seek further training? This is your personal conflict, your realization on meeting the inspiring person that things just weren't right. You resolved this by taking the journey. Resolution does not mean that the issue in question is actually resolved, indeed at your end point you might have more of an appreciation about how unresolved the issue is—but this is a personal resolution in itself, i.e. reaching the personal understanding that there is a bigger problem out there that needs to be fixed, and that you are the person to fix it. Infuse the beginning of your narrative with personal conflict, and conclude the journey with a sense of personal resolution—this makes for a satisfying read, and will give your answer a satisfying sense of self-inclusion for the interviewer. Of course, you must do this authentically, and like with an autobiography the facts must also be truths—this is just a way of you filtering out and structuring the truths from your life and experiences, and a way for you to present these to the interviewer. We are not writing fiction, we a structuring and packaging fact in a way that will make sense to the interviewer, and will thereby draw them towards your humanity. You are a person, not just a number on a list of interview candidates, and however standardized and detached they might try to be, your personal narrative will draw them into the real reason they are there: to find the right person for this job.

Reframing the abstract fact

As a forensic psychiatrist I have often given evidence in court as an expert witness. In the process of this it has often been the case that a cross-examining barrister has tried to extract from me my agreement or disagreement regarding an abstract fact, using words like 'that's right, isn't it … we just need a yes or a no, sir'. I never, or rarely, collude with questions like this, for the simple reason that it is my job as a witness to provide the context behind what might appear to be a simple answer. Rarely in life is the answer ever just yes or no—as dichotomous as the British legal system might be, life does not work in that way, and rather than black and white we find ourselves wading through swathes of grey. Even if the interviewer asks a question that could potentially be answered in just a single word, consider for a moment the context of that question and how you, as a person that wants this job, feel and think about that particular context. I am not suggesting that every potentially simple answer is embellished with a rich and rolling narrative, but I am pointing out that even the simplest of technical questions are still asking a much bigger unsaid question: are you the right person for this job. Therefore, you should use every opportunity to answer that unsaid question and give the interviewer his simple answer, but within a context that includes an essence of you as a person. Do this by reflecting for a moment, and then applying the narrative structure to this simplest of questions, i.e. the beginning, middle, and end of your journey with regards to this particular abstract fact, and the personal conflict and resolution inherent in its material context.

The next exercise will help you to find the narrative within your own field of expertise, and will suggest a method of using a narrative framework to structure your answers in the interview (Exercise 15.1 and Figure 15.1).

EXERCISE 15.1 FINDING THE NARRATIVE

For this exercise research common interview questions within your own field of expertise and list these on a sheet of paper. These might include questions such as: tell me about yourself; what are your strengths and weaknesses; what makes you the right person for this job; how have you demonstrated leadership in your career so far; what motivates you; how have you shown initiative in the past; why this job; why should I hire you; what are your interests and hobbies; are you a team player; have you developed services in the past; tell me about a confrontation with a colleague; tell me about a problem you have solved; how do you deal with stress; how do you respond to a colleague in difficulty; and so on—the list can be a very long one.

Take a fresh sheet of A4 paper and write one of the interview questions at the top of the page (see Figure 15.1). Half way down the page draw a horizontal line from left to right, and label it 'beginning' on the far left and 'end' on the far right. This is your time-line. At the bottom of the page on the left, write the word 'conflict' and circle this. On the right side of the page at the top, diagonally opposite to conflict, write the word 'resolution' and circle this. Draw a diagonal line between these two words—this is your conflict-resolution dimension. Next annotate the page with thoughts, feelings, and facts, as they occur to you. Try to start at the beginning and populate the left side of the page with words and events that come to mind, factual occurrences and their associated thoughts, also the feelings these invoked. Do the same for the middle of the page—your journey towards the present, and on the right consider the end point. Now think of important events that set you out on this journey, the conflicts inherent in that start— again, split these into thoughts, facts, and feelings, and populate the lower left side of the page. Now think about the resolution and do the same. This is your narrative, and once completed you can study the diagram as a whole and think about how you might succinctly answer the question at the top of the page. If it helps, video yourself answering this question for two minutes, as fluently as you can. Watch it back and repeat. Do this for other questions, and develop a method of finding the narrative, your narrative, within your field of expertise.

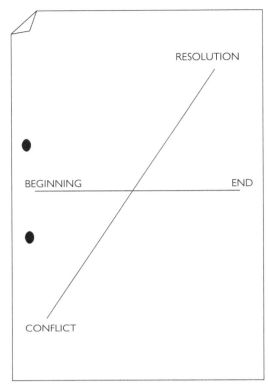

Figure 15.1 Finding the narrative
Find the narrative within your own field of expertise, and use a narrative framework to structure your answers in the interview.

Believing the story

Now that you have found your narrative, you should believe in it. We have worked hard to find an authentic, truthful narrative, and have reframed even the most straightforward of questions into a form that is more human, more about us as people—for this to mean something, we must truly believe in it. This takes us back to the unsaid premise behind any interview question: whatever they are asking, they are only asking it to get an insight into you as a person. Therefore, by reframing facts into a more personal narrative we are answering that unsaid question while also answering the overt said one. It might take a while for you to feel comfortable approaching answers in this way, and like anything it will take time and rehearsal for it to become second nature. You might decide that this approach is not for you, and like any of the suggestions in this book, just use what you find helpful. But whether or not you decide to follow a narrative structure, it is important to believe whatever story you tell the interviewer, since only with your sincere belief is there any chance of the interviewer believing it. Truth is a hard thing to spot and a very difficult thing to discount, but depending on the mood and mental state of the interviewer you could either be lucky or unlucky in this regard. If the interviewer is having a particularly bad day then their threshold for the acceptance of veracity in a candidate may well be higher than if they are feeling happy and relaxed—this is basic human psychology, and however detached and standardized the process might be, we all tend to bias the information we process depending on how we feel in that moment. You must demonstrate your veracity by wholly believing in your own story, and for that reason, your story must therefore be wholly truthful.

Injecting emotion

A critical element in any narrative is emotion, and without this even the most interesting story will appear drab. It may be that you have considered your narrative journey from an emotional perspective as we discussed earlier, but even with this consideration your delivery needs to also be at least partly emotionally driven. We should not be over-emotional, and indeed we need to be especially careful of this when talking through a more personal narrative, but some emotion is required. Emotion needs to be injected into our delivery, it needs to be applied like any of our other skills. This can and should be subtle, but it needs to be there. When you speak of conflict, frown slightly and try to connect with the feelings. Likewise with resolution, relax your face, smile, and connect with the peaceful sense of personal resolution. If you are describing difficult things, employ your empathy skills to communicate this. If the journey is positive then respond in kind. Make your communication congruent with the content, and dig down into your emotions to drive this consistency. Don't be detached and dispassionate as the interviewer may be appearing—be human, draw them from their detached standpoint and into your human narrative. Answer the unsaid question, and show the interviewer that you are the right person for this job.

Skills toolkit 3: Wild cards

Wild cards

There are different kinds of interviews, both structured and unstructured, and many variations in the ways that you can be tested as a candidate. These might include clinical scenarios or work-based tasks, actors as patients, or even written assessments. This book is not concerned with the format of the interview, but more with the underlying psychological processes at play. One such process is the desire of the interviewer to watch you solve a problem live, in front of them. Problem solving is an essential requirement for most jobs, but very difficult to test in a standardized pre-published interview format. Therefore, other components might be used to test this, for example, the clinical patient scenario as a part of standardized medical and surgical training interviews. Whatever the format of the interview, it is likely that you will at some point come across a 'wild card'—this is a question or scenario that you have not prepared for, and by its very nature it will be challenging and very discriminating between different interview candidates. In this chapter we will consider some generic psychological strategies for dealing with wild cards, and will work together to try to overcome this particular challenging interview hurdle.

Facing the unknown

Facing the unknown is terrifying, there is no easier way of putting it. Especially in an important job interview, one that might impact significantly upon your future career and earning—the unknown interview component is a variable over which we have no control, and this can feel unbearable in the weeks and days before the interview. The more we work towards stifling our anxiety by over-learning questions that are sure to come up, the more we will be overcome by anxiety when faced with the surety of the unknown interview component. Of course, in this book we do not over-learn, indeed we embrace interview anxiety so already are in a relatively stronger starting position when it comes to facing the unknown. But regardless, this is a difficult part of the interview process, both pragmatically and psychologically, and in this chapter we will try to overcome this difficulty.

The first step is accepting the fact that the unknown is terrifying for everyone, and all candidates will struggle with this particular hurdle. In some ways, the wild card is the fairest interview component since no one can really prepare for it. We are all in the same boat, and must all just do whatever we can to get past this. The wild card will test our problem-solving skills in a novel way, and all we can do is apply those skills carefully and methodically. The approach in this book of being mindful and connected wholly with the interview experience is particularly relevant during the wild card component, since being connected with this particular task and focussing all available resources to it is essential. There are no learnt answers or scenarios that can help us with this, all we can do is be entirely connected with the task of solving the problem during that actual moment.

Reacting and adapting

If you've ever sat on the edge of your seat during a horror movie, you know how unsettling and terrifying the unknown can be—that sense of impending doom and dread. However, if instead of anxiously squirming and biting your hand in anticipation, you relax back in the chair and force yourself to breathe normally, you relax your arms and hands, and just surrender yourself to the moment, to the unknown—then you will be less terrified. Try it. This is a basic psychological response, and it's rather like forcing yourself to smile when you feel flat—the smile will make you feel better. You need to relax into the unknown and surrender to the uncertainty, adopt a mindful connected state throughout your interview, and force yourself back to this tonic position of connection when faced with uncertainty. Don't allow fear to creep in and distort your perceptions and abilities—you should operate calmly and in complete control of your skills and faculties.

Consider the way that you react to the wild card in your interview from the perspective of the interviewer—think about the fact that firstly, they expect this to be new and unknown to you, and secondly, the way you react is actually part of the test here. The whole point of an unknown scenario like this is to test your reaction to a new and novel problem, and to see how you solve it. Sometimes the problem will be unsolvable, sometimes there may not be only one right answer— these are the best kinds of wild cards since they push your behaviours and acumen to the limit. Herein lies a comforting thought regarding wild cards—absolve yourself of the underlying belief that there is a right answer, and simply consider what you think a possible answer to this problem might be. This is a situation in life where the journey is most definitely more important than the final destination, and whilst they might prefer you to reach the 'right' conclusion, more often than not most of the potential marks for the interview will be gathered along the journey. They will be specifically interested in the way you react and adapt to the unknown, and will be looking for a calm, logical, and measured approach, utilizing all of your skills and acumen—focus on this rather than the final destination, and make sure that your journey to the end-point demonstrates your abilities to the fullest.

In fact, a wild card in your interview is a fantastic opportunity to shine, it is a rare moment when most candidates will be on a level playing field, and you can also utilize a core skill inherent in all of us as humans: curiosity in the face of something novel. Toddlers will naturally explore their environment with curiosity, and most of us enjoy this basic human behaviour throughout our life. The interview raises the stakes and can make what might have been a fun task seem impossible— but perhaps it will appear impossible to all candidates, and perhaps a good approach to the novel problem should be with child-like curiosity and interest. Apply yourself to the task with vigour and enthusiasm, don't let any fear or trepidation sneak through your armour of composure and control—employ your non-technical skills and relax into the task. After all, it is likely that this task will mirror the kind of task that would be commonplace were you to be successful in this interview and get the job, so approach the task accordingly. If the wild card is a question then use the same skills and apply yourself with vigour and curiosity. If you are surprised by the task and question, then show that—be honest and authentic in your response, just don't let fear and trepidation give the wrong impression of you as a candidate. You need to rise to the challenge of the unknown, and tackle it as you would were you to be an employee.

During the course of the wild card component of the interview you will be problem-solving live, in front of the interviewer, whether performing a difficult task or formulating a challenging answer. Treat this as you would an A-level maths problem, when the examiner wants to see your workings as well as the final answer. The working tells so much about your process, and the way that you might react in other challenging scenarios, so show it. It is a bit like doing your driving test, when you want to demonstrate clearly to the test instructor that you are indeed checking in the rear-view mirror. They need to see you actually do that. Use some of the skills we have previously discussed, such as signposting, to make your thinking and problem-solving process very clear. Sometimes the direction of travel, i.e. the pathway of a line of questioning of a patient, or a particular method in solving a task, is more important than the specific questions or skills—make sure the interviewer can see your compass heading. Don't, however, break the illusion of the test. The wild card is essentially a simulation of a novel problem you might typically face at work, and its strength as a disseminating interview task depends partly on its ability to simulate real life as closely as possible. Inherent in this is a willing suspension of disbelief from yourself and the interviewer, and your approach to the task should be as though you were doing this in the real world rather than just the interview.

The ability to adapt to new situations in life is a core tenet for survival, and adaptation is critical for success in the wild card component of the interview, be it a task, scenario, or question. Adaptation requires cognitive and emotional flexibility, moving out of our normal trenches and pathways of behaviour, and into the unknown. Adaptation in itself may be a core skill the interviewer is looking for, depending on the nature of the problem—but whether it is a specific point to score or not, it is a commendable attribute to demonstrate. Be panoramic in your approach to the problem, and as best as you can, think outside of the box. It is unlikely that the problem will just require a rote-learned pattern of thinking or behaviour, but even if this is the case use the problem as an opportunity to flourish and shine. Demonstrate your adaptability to adapt and change your methods during novel and challenging situations, and overtly signpost your methods of adaptation. This might be by using different strategies with a difficult unresponsive patient in order to get them to engage with you, or could be by employing a few different techniques in solving a task. The importance is in your approach being one of adaptation, rather than trying to use your normal comfortable pre-learnt patterns of behaviour—you can be grounded by a bedrock of learned behaviours, but use these as your foundations rather than the whole building. The building should be constructed with your adaptability, problem-solving skills, and innovative ideas, built upon a bedrock of stability. Adapt to the unknown in your interview, and thereby show the interviewer that you can potentially adapt to anything.

The following exercise will help you deal with wild cards in your interview (Exercise 16.1).

EXERCISE 16.1 DEALING WITH WILD CARDS

The premise for this exercise is the notion that whatever unknown scenarios you might face in your interview, these will mirror real-world problems that you are already solving day-in and day-out. The wild card is a simulation of common problems within your own profession or specialty, and although they may differ and be more advanced given that they will reflect problems you might face in your new role should you be successful in getting the job, they will probably be similar to the problems you already deal with regularly. Even if the wild card in the interview is markedly different to any problem you have previously dealt with, the technique in this exercise will still be useful to you, since it involves mindfully deconstructing your problem-solving skills in day-to-day tasks, and thereby creating a framework you can apply to new situations in the interview.

When you are faced with a challenging problem at work, in the weeks and days prior to your interview, try to assume a more objective standpoint and be an observer of your own actions.

(continued)

You can still focus on the task, but allow yourself the luxury of also standing back and considering your actions and behaviours from a more objective position, be an investigator of your own problem-solving skills. Consider the way you react to the problem, how it makes you feel and the thoughts that run through your head. If possible, write these down, if not right now then later. Think about how you need to adapt your skills to solve this problem, be it a task or conversation with a relative—whatever the situation, overtly try to break down your process of adaptation in a way you could describe to a friend. If you act on instinct alone, then try to delve into this and work out what actually happened, what were the thoughts and inspirations behind your new strategy.

Either at the time or later, document the process on a new page of a note book—list the problem, and add any contextual factors that will take you back to the situation, e.g. time, date, location. Document the thoughts, feelings, and facts. Think about the narrative—draw a timeline, then add a diagonal line to represent the conflict-resolution dimension. Populate the page with words, and repeat this process every time you are faced with a novel problem. In time you will notice patterns starting to form. Then, in your interview, you will have a visual memory of the strategies you have employed to problem-solve in the past—structure your mind in this way, start at the beginning, and resolve whatever conflict exists.

Discover your edge

During the process of problem solving, especially in novel situations, you will have discovered aspects of your personality and skillset that make you especially good in this particular task. We are all unique, and whatever the problem in life we all bring our unique qualities to solve it. Even if a novel problem in the interview has only one correct solution there will be many different ways to get to that end-point, and you will be marked on the journey itself. What are the particular aspects of you, as a person, that make you successful in solving problems? Perhaps you are more of a people-person, who finds inter-relational ways of solving problems. Perhaps you are more technically minded, and are able to block out the rest of the world as you focus on the wires and switches. Whatever your strength, this is unique to you and will appear so in the interview. This is your edge, and whilst other candidates will also have strengths, theirs will be different to yours. It is useful to embrace our particular strengths and recognize them as a unique edge. This is your access point to success in this part of the interview, the keyhole in the locked door of the novel problem. You shouldn't depend wholly on your edge, but it might be a good starting point, or at least a good default to fall back on if things appear impossible. Even if you don't manage to solve the problem, at least let the interviewer know what it is about you that is unique. With a good understanding and acceptance of the value of your own unique qualities, the interviewer will be more likely to discover your edge for themselves.

Endings and closure

We will consider the importance of endings and closure later in this book (see Chapter 19), but for now think of the wild card scenario as a self-contained aspect of the interview. This may be the only place that the interviewer gets to see you problem-solve live in front of them, and is potentially testing very different skills to those tested in the rest of the interview. Therefore, this part of the interview should have its own sense of closure. Furthermore, a problem-solving task, whether an unknown question or patient interview, needs to have an ending—we would hope that the ending is the resolution of the problem, but it is important that you demonstrate personal closure and resolution even if you have not been able to complete the task successfully. It is helpful to convey to the interviewer your insight into the end of this task, whether or not it has gone well. If you have been successful then the resolution is inbuilt, but without success you need to try to convey a sense of your insight into failure, and that you are resolved in the fact that you could not complete the task today. Insight into failure gives the interviewer a strong sense that you might be successful in the future, whereas a lack of insight just says that the whole thing is beyond your comprehension. Knowing that something was just too difficult is better than not knowing anything at all.

The final reason for a sense of personal closure after a challenging task is to protect yourself from dangerous after-flow effects, i.e. the risk that performing badly in this task might make you more likely to perform badly in those that follow. If you are not successful in the wild card component you just need to move on, realizing that perhaps others have found it just as hard, and with the objective of not contaminating the rest of the interview with this failure. A good way to move on is to overtly end the scenario with the interviewer, either with a few words or even non-verbal cues, so that you both know that you have absolute insight into the difficulty of this task, and also implicitly implying that you might be successful next time. You don't actually say that, by the way, you just imply it. Closure will help to resolve the conflict this problem has created in you, even if that closure is essentially overtly accepting defeat in the eyes of the interviewer. Then, move on, and leave this challenging task behind you.

Skills toolkit 4: The non-technical expert

Soft skills

Almost every interview will have a pre-set marking pattern that is transparent and available for close scrutiny should a candidate complain that the process was biased, discriminatory, or unfair. Some interviews are standardized to the point that the interviewer is no longer allowed to ask what they like, instead they need to read from a laminated sheet, the same sheet that has been available to the candidate for a month before. This is the world we live in. So in this era of transparency and standardization, where is the room for an interviewer to follow their gut and hire the person they instinctually feel is the right person? Does this still happen? I would suggest that it does, indeed it must, since the process of choosing candidates is beyond just the overt questions and answers—it is based on much more nebulous factors present in the room. The presence of the candidate, their attitude and professionalism, the way they process and react, their overall manner—these things are hard to score on a sheet but have massive potential impact in the selection process. These are our soft skills, and their impact is substantial. As an analogy, think of a driving test—the test instructor has to pass or fail candidates according to their score sheet, but what really happens is they either feel safe when you drive or they don't. This is based on aspects of your performance not easily collected on a score sheet, but is a strong influence that will guide their decision-making process, as it should. In this chapter we will consider our non-technical skills, our soft skills, as they pertain to the interview.

Survival mode

During high-pressure stressful situations when we a forced to problem-solve, and are functioning at the limits of our intellectual capacity, our soft skills tend to fall away as we preserve our energy for what appears to be more important. In survival mode we focus on the essential and tend to neglect what appears to be superfluous. Even if we value soft skills such as eye contact and empathy, it is difficult to maintain these in the face of stress and adversity. To do so requires active application, and whilst such skills need to trundle along in the background passively rather than requiring conscious thought, to achieve this state takes practice within a framework of psychological understanding. We know that the interviewer's impression of us will be guided by not only what we say but the way that we say it, the way we come across—and with this understanding we should rehearse our soft skills every time we interact socially between now and the interview. The interview will push you into survival mode, but don't let it strip you of a wealth of skills that can function happily in the background, and that will improve your presence in the eyes of the interviewer.

Eye contact and touch

From a psychological perspective there is a space between you and the interviewer, and many of your non-technical skills are acting to reduce that space. Eye contact and physical touch are examples of these. As a recent interviewer myself, I can speak to my own discomfort and annoyance at a stream of candidates having no apparent consideration or respect for my own personal psychological space—they mostly all shook my hand and stared directly at me, as though they had been trained to do that with no psychological understanding of what they were actually doing. Any interview guide will tell you to make eye contact with the interviewer, and indeed this is essential—but be aware that by making eye contact you are entering the interviewer's psychological space, and so it might be appropriate to do this thoughtfully rather than absolutely, and to glance around the interviewer in a natural way as the interaction progresses. If you were to meet a friend it would be strange to stare fixedly at them the entire time—there is normally an interplay of eye contact, where both people fix and unfix contact as the conversation warrants. Try to be natural with eye contact, and look at the spot between the eyebrows rather than directly into the eyes. Also, break eye contact occasionally, perhaps as you reflect before answering a question, and give the interviewer the chance to feel comfortable in their own observations of you.

Regarding handshakes or other physical contact, I personally would never do this, but perhaps that's just me. I would not mark a candidate down if they insisted on shaking my hand, but I find it rather intrusive and really don't understand why any interview guidance would instruct candidates to shake hands as a standard. If your business or profession does expect a handshake then do so, but be mindful of the interviewer's space and do not be overbearing. Apply some pressure, but try to modulate the pressure depending on the shake of the interviewer. Whatever you choose, just be mindful of the psychological underpinnings at play in the room.

Warmth and professionalism

Warmth and affability are excellent qualities in an interview candidate, and you should strive for this in your interview. Don't be put off if the interviewer appears cold and detached—this does not reflect on you as a person, and you should not take such an attitude personally. Just be warm, as you might be to a customer or patient, and be the kind of person they might naturally warm to. This should be balanced with your professionalism though, and you should be aware of this potential conflict. Professionalism is colder and more calculated, precise and objective—it works hand-in-hand with warmth and your humanity, but the two states can be difficult to get exactly right. I suggest starting from a position of warmth, then retreating to a more objective professional standpoint when you are asked questions. Think of yourself moving between the two positions, rather than trying to be both at once. You want to appear human, and to do this you must dial up and dial down your warmth, as you replace that stance with a more professional one. Try to vacillate between these two states in rehearsal, then find a subtle version of that for the interview itself.

Empathy and distance

We have considered empathy and connection with the interviewer in detail already (see Chapter 5) but here I take you back to the idea of space between you and the interviewer, and the concept that your non-technical skills are acting to pull you both closer together. Empathy communicates your humanity to the interviewer and it is a powerful way for you to both express and read nuanced social cues and communications. Empathy pulls you closer together, but in your interview you should balance this with a slight increase in distance between you and the interviewer should that be appropriate. This is a balance, and you can modulate the distance between you by either dialling up or dialling down the tone and intensity of your empathy. How and when to do this depends on the interview itself, but as a rule you should dial up the empathy when you want to overtly demonstrate compassion, understanding, and humanity, and pull back when you want to be more authoritarian, paternalistic, and professional. For example, if you were to discuss sick patients you would dial up the empathy, but if you went on to discuss a new treatment strategy you might dial back on the empathy and increase the distance, taking a more professional and objective standpoint. If you are in the wild card part of the interview speaking to a patient, you might dial up empathy as you connect on a human level but then dial back as you become subtly paternalistic and encourage them to feel hopeful about a new treatment option. The exact nature of the empathy and distance between you both will depend on your specific profession and specialty, but the psychological underpinnings are the same. Use it to your advantage, and let the interviewer see that you are not only human, but that you can also be a rock of stability for other humans.

Confidence and humility

Confidence, unless truly earned and believed in, is a fragile, translucent sheet of glass that can be easily cracked in the interview. Of course, we should all be confident, but to just give that advice is similar to telling a person not to be afraid when they are terrified. A candidate who is wholly confident appears either unconvincing or overly so—in reality, a truly confident person will feel more and less confident about aspects of themselves and their performance, and this modulation should occur throughout the interview. Know your edge and feel confident about it, but don't wear a fragile defence of insincere confidence as this will be seen through immediately. Your confidence should be balanced by your sense of humility—don't be self-deprecating, but be humble. Move between these two positions. In that way, your confidence will appear more authentic when strategically placed next to your humility.

Body language and the non-verbal

We covered this in detail in Chapter 11, but I will mention a few things here for the sake of completeness. Be aware of your physical presence in the room, and the way that this contributes to the space as a whole. Don't be self-conscious, just be self-aware from a psychological perspective, and understand the impact that your body language and non-verbal communications have on the interviewer. Assume a comfortable and relaxed tonic position, don't use any superfluous body movements and try not to fidget. Centre yourself in the chair, in the room, and be mindful of your surroundings—be connected to the moment, here and now, and understand how your physical presence influences that moment. Consider the space created for you in the room and fill the required space, not too much and not too little. Think of your body language adding to any speech to fill the space and don't over-fill or be too overbearing. Use your body language and non-verbal communications to annotate your expression overall, but do this in a subtle way. Don't forget facial expression, and aim for a state of physical congruence between what you say and the way you come across to the interviewer. Your body language is an extension of yourself as a person—use it to answer the unsaid question: is this the right person for this job? Be that person.

Your body language and physical presence is your interface with the world around you. It is just as important and powerful as the words you say. Being aware of this in itself should be helpful, since it gives you the potential to tap into an extremely powerful and effective resource readily available to you. Consider your physical presence in every interaction between now and your interview; modulate the subtleties of your performance to the outside world so that your true authentic self is reflected. The authentic you isn't anxious and neurotic, your anxiety and neuroses result from the interview process. They are necessary by-products of this charged psychological encounter. Package them away, and present yourself to the world as the best you can be (see Box 17.1).

BOX 17.1 **ANECDOTE**

Don't forget to smile ...

Good advice for any interview candidate.

Reflection: In stressful situations it is hard to smile, since doing so requires a lightness of spirit and confidence that is almost unreachable while we focus wholly on solving the problem at hand. Herein lies the strength of a smile, because doing so implies that we are light of spirit, that we are confident, and that we can take this interview in our stride and retain our humour and humanity. Also, smiling on the outside tends to make us smile on the inside.

Friends and colleagues

Being friendly is clearly not the same as being a friend, but both things emerge from the same place: a human desire for social connection and acceptance. The interviewer is not your friend and may never be, but if you were to get this job then the potential for friendship should at least be on the table, and you must certainly be a friendly candidate. This is balanced with a more collegiate position, where mutual respect overrides the basic need for connection and acceptance. Hold both positions in your mind—they are both important but not easily established concurrently. Move between the two positions and make the interviewer aware that whilst you are friendly in nature, you are in essence a respectful colleague. Inherent in this is an understanding of space and psychological boundaries, and you should have a good understanding of this as an interview candidate. Many work environments require solid boundaries, and whilst things can be friendlier around the water-cooler, a more distanced position may be needed in the office. Demonstrate your flexibility in this, underpinned by your appreciation of the need for psychological boundaries at work. Do this by moving between the position of friend and colleague as the interview progresses.

Insight

During the interview, and in the days and weeks before, it is important to have a robust insight into your strengths, weaknesses, and mental state. If you perform well, or not so well, in the interview then this information should be known to you—self-monitoring of performance is essential for your optimization and improvement. Insight is only possible if you truly see yourself, the good and the bad, free from defences and self-deceptions. It's no use blindly telling yourself that everything is fine—you need to know exactly how things are going, and this requires brutal self-honesty. Self-monitoring is a process that should occur throughout the whole interview process, and indeed your ability to self-monitor may be of interest to the interviewer. Insight into your strengths and weaknesses may also be required for dissemination in the interview room, but knowledge of these is also critical for your own internal checks and balances. Keep your eyes open, to the room and to yourself, and don't allow a shroud of self-deception even if this might make you feel better in the short-term—always choose undefended honesty, and retain full insight throughout this process.

The capacity for change

Demonstrate to the interviewer your capacity for change, your ability to process the environment, and adapt as required—this can be shown live, in the actual room, and also disseminated in the examples you give about your journey, and your plans and aspirations for the future. Change is always good, never settle for comfortable stagnancy. Stand firm with your beliefs and convictions, even stick with some opinion and conjecture, but allow these to guide change in your practice and performance. Find the conflict between your ideals and the world around you, and instigate change to resolve that discrepancy.

CHAPTER 18

Generic approach 1: Modular, dynamic skills

A modular, dynamic skillset

Adopting a generic approach to the interview allows skills to be seamlessly transferred between different questions and tasks, and improves the chance of success in unexpected aspects of the process—but this should be balanced with good preparation of specific content that is likely to be relevant in your given profession and specialty. I suggest that it is useful to adopt a generic approach, the intention being that this is a psychologically driven strategy that underpins the whole interview, and upon this can be attached more specific content-driven aspects of preparation and performance. As well as the potential for improved performance in the interview, a generic approach also improves our ability to learn from mistakes and inform our future attempts—this is because we make efforts to break down our experience into core building blocks, and these can be slotted into existing skillsets regardless of the specific context in which they were learnt. Our skills should be thought of as modular and dynamic, as should our digestion and processing of our interview experiences. In this way, although an interview is an essentially summative experience, providing us with a timestamp of our abilities, we can transform the experience into a formative one that can potentially improve our future attempts.

We have previously discussed a process of transforming contextually learnt experiences into modular threads and skills (see Chapter 14) and we can employ a similar process here, by extracting building blocks and assigning them with psychological power in the form of thoughts and feelings (see Exercise 14.1: Constructing modular threads, Chapter 14). The idea is that a skill is made up of core psychological facets, and that these can be used in other questions and situations; whereas the skill in its original form may be less transferable and useful elsewhere. Skills should be modular and dynamic, not contextual and static. Indeed, once a skill has been acquired it can be both dynamically applied and also improved upon—every time a skill is used in different situations it can be refined and optimized. Of course, many skills will already transfer across easily—this is just a method of breaking things down psychologically and packaging the skills in a more transferrable way. How you choose to hold your skills in mind in a more modular dynamic form is entirely up to you—the important thing is that they are modular and dynamic, rather than static and fixed to a particular context.

Application and processes

Application of a dynamic skillset requires flexibility of thinking and adaptation during the interview, and whilst this approach does not give us a sense of security walking into the room since we are not armoured up with pre-set patterns of behaviour, it does give us the ability to adapt our performance and make it exactly the right fit for purpose. Adaptation allows us to refine our performance, and with good insight and self-monitoring we can reach much higher levels of expertise than we might do otherwise. Consider a challenging and novel question in the interview—as candidates we would fall back on our core strengths and qualities to overcome this, such strengths tend to be nebulous and relatable in most situations. We might also have access to skills applicable in this situation. But now, with our modular dynamic skillset, we can select more specific skills driven by and imbued with core psychological strengths and qualities, and by applying these we can add refinement to our problem-solving strategies.

We have thought about several different psychological approaches and processes in this book, and these have all been generic at their core. We have considered the room to be divided into the concrete, the material, and the abstract. We have thought about building blocks of thought, feeling, and fact. We have considered narrative structure as a way of conceptualizing journeys and even abstract facts. We are armed with a wealth of psychological processes, and with these as our scaffolding we can move forward in any task utilizing our dynamic skillset as we need. We are equipped with a psychological framework of understanding, and along with our modular threads and dynamic skills, we can adapt and mould ourselves to fit any situation in the interview. This should give us confidence and hope, and doesn't at all take away from any of the specific content-driven preparation we might have done for the interview, either in our groups or from our previous interview experiences. We have the full package.

In Exercise 18.1 we will consider the value of being cognitively flexible in the interview.

EXERCISE 18.1 **BENDING IN THE WIND**

I once left court after giving evidence and had a drink with the barrister. I told him I was worried I had been too flexible in my stance on the stand, and that I had conceded too much in cross-examination. He told me to stay flexible, that flexibility was a key quality of mine. He said that rigid and brittle expert witnesses are easily broken by the opposing counsel. It is rather like a willow tree that bends in the wind, or an earthquake-proof building that actually sways and moves with the vibrations. Flexibility is key, in many parts of life, and in the interview. Flexibility of thought can be a formidable quality in the interview—not by conceding and acquiescing to someone else's opinion, but by reflecting and re-evaluating the evidence so that your thoughts and opinions can adapt live in front of the interviewer. In that way, you demonstrate the potential for growth in the future, the ability to learn, and also a remarkable strength of character. In this exercise we will work on actively trying to change a thought or opinion, as an active applied psychological process, and thereby rehearse this important potential core generic quality for your interview.

At school you may or may not have had the experience of being a member of the debating team, but here we will do something similar. The objective is to pick a current affair you feel strongly about and argue the case for the other side, the opposing counsel as it were. It has to be something that has emotional impact for you, maybe even something with personal ramifications that has in some way directly affected a friend or family member. The best subject matter is something that makes you feel very angry or upset, ideally to the point of fury or tears—and given the state of the world, I'm sure there are plenty of subjects to choose from. On a piece of A4 paper write the subject matter, in a sentence, at the top of the page. Under this, write a sentence or two that captures your thoughts on this matter, something unique to

(continued)

you, an individual angle or perspective that captures your position. Draw a horizontal line under this, and another one dividing the lower section into two halves, upper and lower.

Label the section below 'opposing counsel', and divide this middle part of the page into three columns. Label the columns 'fact', 'feelings', and 'thoughts'. Next research this subject matter on the internet, and search for facts that back up the contrary view to your own—list key words that represent these facts in the first column. Spend time on the research and really try to see the argument from the other side. Put yourself in the shoes of the other side and try to connect with the way they feel. Absorb those feelings, and write key feelings down in the second column. Next reflect on these facts and feelings, try to emotionally connect with them and don't feel conflicted by your initial belief or personal investment in this matter—this is just a psychological experiment. You are allowed to embrace the contrary argument here. Indeed, you are encouraged to. Finally, write a sentence in the lower section that captures this new opposing position—the kind of statement opposing counsel might make, and one that balances the initial statement you wrote at the top of the paper.

Reflect on these two positions, and consider how reflecting on opposing facts and feelings led you to consider new thoughts and opinions. Of course, you will probably still hold your previous view, and your thoughts and opinions may not have changed at all—but by repeating this exercise and applying yourself to the task, you will be re-treading a psychological pathway to flexibility of thought and potential change.

Reading the reflections

We have considered the value of adaptation and flexibility in formulating answers to questions in the interview, and have been closely monitoring our performance in order to optimize these changes. We have also considered our dynamic modular skills and how these, driven by and constructed upon core psychological facets and processes, can be applied adaptively in our interview. There is another powerful source of information in the interview, beyond our own insights and monitoring, beyond our reading of the material and abstract elements in the room—this other source of information is located in your interviewer. In fact, the interviewer is our collaborator in this charged psychological interaction, they are our co-conspirators in this endeavour. This is because firstly, they are human, with their own set of non-verbal communications and physical tells, ripe for reading, and perfect for informing our flexible approach and adaptive performance. Secondly, it is likely that the interviewer will be rooting for you, especially if you can demonstrate your humanity through your warmth and empathy alongside your aptitude, and whilst they will not give you an unfair advantage they will probably act in ways that can potentially facilitate your performance. An interviewer wants to get the best out of a candidate, they want to see the best in that candidate, and being human themselves they will encourage and facilitate this as best they can. Of course, it is possible that you may come across an interviewer who is not at all encouraging, indeed some can appear the exact opposite—but we will start from a more positive position, since only by looking will we have any hope of finding interviewer collaboration and facilitation.

As part of your process in connecting to the room and this moment, you must pay particular attention to the interviewer—their facial expressions, body language, and empathy, nothing should be missed. We have considered the interview from their perspective and have discussed theory of mind, but alongside this theoretical construct about what they might be thinking, let us carefully pick up any clues as to what they are actually thinking. This might be in the form of the slightest of smiles, or a nod of encouragement. It might be a more animated body language when things are going well, and a more closed off position when things are going badly. Read this body language carefully, pick up on all the potential cues and modify your performance accordingly. Aim to increase the times when the interviewer seems happy with your performance, and minimize the times when they are more shut down. Let them lead you subtly through this process, and if they are giving the right cues, be guided by them toward success. This isn't a rule set in stone and you should follow them with care, but being guided by their non-verbal communications and body language could be very helpful, and if they are the kind of person to deliberately mislead you then this really isn't the kind of place you'd like to work anyway.

To practice this, in the days and weeks before your interview, try to overtly pick up on colleagues' body language and non-verbal communications and adapt accordingly—no longer will you just think about what you will be saying next; from now on really concentrate on what they are saying, how they are saying it, and what their body is telling you. Engage in the non-verbal, and learn a whole new way of communicating and reacting to the world around you.

It is much harder, if not impossible, to read the reflections if you are conducting an online or video interview, but even in this situation an awareness of the interviewers' body language and presence is still important. Given the importance of cues in the room it could be that you are at a disadvantage if you interview online, but don't let this concern you as there are pros and cons to this situation. You can't easily read the room on a video screen, but on the other hand it is easier for you to control the way you come across to the interviewer since all they see is what you present to them on screen. Given a choice, attend in person if you can, but don't let an online or video interview erode your confidence (see Box 18.1).

BOX 18.1 **ANECDOTE**

Online or video interviews are always a challenge, but they can work ...

Thoughts on the remote interview.

Reflection: It is always better to appear in person, but if you absolutely have to interview remotely then this can still lead to success. Prepare in the same way you would a normal interview, including your attire, and also test your internet connection or video conferencing to make sure the picture and audio is clear. Check your image on the screen and arrange the wall behind you so the impression is professional and uncluttered. Try to sit far enough back so the interviewer can see your whole upper body, rather than just your head and shoulders—they need to see your body language. Rehearse speaking and film your performance—you need to gauge and modulate the degree of your body movements until they have impact on a computer screen, and this might mean being more effusive than you might be in person. The objective is to be able to communicate to the interviewer verbally and non-verbally, just as effectively as though you were in the room. Also, make extra effort in trying to read the interviewer's body language, and be partly guided by this in your performance.

CHAPTER 19

Generic approach 2: Generic templates

CONTENTS

A generic template

We have spent much of this book considering different frameworks of psychological understanding, and here at the end we will discuss a more concrete framework: a generic template you can use to help guide you through each stage of the interview. This generic template has five simple steps, and I will describe each of these in turn in the following sections of this chapter. You can adapt these and use them as you wish, but I hope they provide you with a starting point should you wish to try to structure your approach to the interview in this way. Of course, this template should not neglect all the previous psychological constructs and processes we have been discussing and developing so far, indeed its success is dependent upon these. This is just a generic approach you can adopt in any interview question or task, and within each step you should employ all the modular and dynamic skills at your disposal.

Focal problem

This is your starting point—what is the interviewer actually asking of you? What is the question? If you are not clear, ask them to repeat it. Reflect for a moment—are you sure you understand what they really want from you in this part of the interview? What is the focal problem? The focal problem might not be the overt question they are asking, or it might be plainly laid out for you to see. The interviewer is not trying to trick you, but just be clear about what they actually want. For example, if they ask you to describe examples when you have been involved in service innovations, then what they are really interested in is how you might be able to innovate services within this role should you be successful—therefore, consider examples that are relevant for this post, rather than any random innovations you might have been involved with. Or if they ask you to talk about a time when you demonstrated leadership, then consider the leadership role required for this particular post and deliver an example accordingly. You should be truthful and authentic, but try to mould your responses in a way that answers the focal problem they have put to you.

Casting a wider net

As you are embarking on your journey and are starting to answer the focal problem, retain a degree of anxiety about your destination and try to gather more information in order to calculate your final compass setting. Do this by speaking slightly around the focal problem and carefully monitoring the response of the interviewer. If you have been set a specific task, don't just launch yourself forwards into that task blindly with no consideration of a change in direction—instead, set off tentatively and reflectively, checking the interviewer carefully for any physical tells that might inform you. Are you travelling in the right direction? It would be a very cruel interviewer who would let a candidate blunder off in the completely the wrong direction without some subtle cues, and if you check carefully you will see these. You might want to ask a clarifying question, to reassure yourself that you are going in the right direction. Once you are sure, then fix your compass setting and start to move forwards through the task.

Moving forwards

Being mindful that any answer should be brief and concise, no longer than a couple of minutes, start to move forwards through the problem. By now you are sure of what the problem actually is, and have checked for any nuances you might have missed—now is the time to employ all of your skills in delivering on this issue. Don't forget to carry on monitoring yourself and the interviewer, and retain a sense of adaptation and flexibility if needed—but here you are essentially disseminating your thoughts and beliefs in a way that is understandable to the interviewer. Perhaps you are using a narrative framework to structure your response. Work your way forwards through the task, steadily and calmly, in a way that is both structured and understood by the interviewer. Be methodical and logical, but don't neglect your warmth and empathy. Be human and pull the interviewer towards you, across the gulf that divides you.

Showing your cards

This is almost the end of the task, but not quite. Here you are reaching your final destination and are demonstrating the starting point of resolution to the interviewer, but you do so with care and monitoring. Does the interviewer want more from you? Read their body language very carefully at this point—if you have been brief and concise there is still time to pull this around if you were wrong. Don't just turn over your cards and drop them onto the table—give yourself the space to rethink and find totally different cards if you need to. For example, in your example about a service innovation, does the interviewer seem satisfied? Are they nodding and preparing the next question, or looking rather pensive and not appearing to move on? Read the non-verbal cues and make your decision. It is no too late to move back slightly and take a different direction, it is never too late to have another try. It is better to be at the bottom of a ladder facing the right direction than at the top of a ladder facing the wrong way. When you are satisfied that this is the final destination, show your cards.

Finding resolution

This is the final part of the task and a critical one. Resolution is essential for your future tasks, as it ensures that however this one went, it is finished and will not bleed into anything that comes next. This is important whether the task or question has gone well or badly—if it went well, then a sense of relief and confidence might skew the next question just as much as if it went badly. The task needs to end, and finding resolution is your way of ensuring that. Resolution might be successful completion then moving on, or it might be you overtly acknowledging that this didn't go well. Don't just leave a task hanging—ensure that you finish it. Then move on.

At the end of the interview resolution is found, for both you and the interviewer, by the very last question: 'do you have any questions for us?' (see Box 19.1).

BOX 19.1 **ANECDOTE**

I always wait for the questions a candidate asks. It usually tells you a lot ...

Some thoughts on the inevitable end-of-interview final task—asking an interesting and relevant question of the interviewer or panel.

Reflection: The question you ask at the end of the interview is an element of your performance that should be researched, ready, and rehearsed. It doesn't need to be unique or ground breaking, but it does need to be relevant and should reflect your enthusiasm for the job, combined with some prior knowledge that you just need slightly elucidating. The interviewer will not necessarily assign marks or kudos depending on the questions you ask, but should you find yourself neck-and-neck with another candidate it would be good to have done everything you could. Consider also what your question tells the interviewer about you, and leave them with the best possible impression.

Final thoughts

CONTENTS

Moving on

The ability to move on is essential for interview success, both in the long and short-term. In the long-term we must learn from our mistakes and grow stronger with each attempt, we must be empowered with every setback and assimilate each experience for the greater good—this is only possible if we can move on from the disappointment of failure. Likewise in the short-term, during the interview itself, we need to let adversity fall away from us and just move on to the next task. Nothing can be allowed to contaminate the process, and an interview task should never be tarnished because of a previous experience—every experience in the interview, good and bad, should be contributing towards improving our future performance. We can achieve this with a strong and robust psychological framework of understanding, underpinning and driving our attitudes and behaviours, informing us and bringing us to a higher level of operation. With work and understanding we can move on after anything, and with every new experience, good and bad, we will only improve.

Embracing the positive

As I contemplate this section I am struck by the lack of mention of positivity previously in this book, and certainly a vacuum of embracing that positivity. So far we have been more minded to embrace anxiety, and to exist in an authentic position where weakness and adversity is seen and acknowledged, not pushed aside for the sake of positivity. But here, in these final thoughts, we will spend a moment reflecting on the positive. The interview is stressful and tends to push us into darker, more difficult places—but we must balance this with positivity. This whole book has been about balance. By embracing the negative we are also able to embrace the positive, and despite the fact that we have left this until just here at the very end, it is never too late to grab hold of positivity and pull it into your life and practice. The building blocks must be real and must be grounded in all those difficult aspects of the interview that we have been discussing so far—but once the foundations are laid and the psychological work has been done, we can drift around in more positive waters and be proud of our work and achievements. Always look for balance—just concentrate on dealing with the negative aspects before you bask in the positive.

Upgrading as appropriate

Every interview is an upgrade, however it turns out. I hope this book has in part been an upgrade, or at least given you a slight change in perspective. If you need to upgrade further then do so. Success in the interview is critical for all of us to move forward in life, and you should be performing at your absolute best in this charged and challenging psychological encounter. Read widely, rehearse, take courses, ask for guidance—do what you can to effect change. Never settle for anything less than your absolute best, and if something is stopping you do that, fix it.

Version 2.0

So here we are, at the end of this book. I hope that you have found it useful. If it has changed anything in your interview practice and performance then that is great, though clearly you have done all the hard work yourself—this book was merely a conduit for your success. Now that you have changed things, you should embrace the opportunity that is the interview. Now that you are a new version, take chances and put yourself out there, surrender to the experience of the interview and connect wholly with that process. The more you do, the better you will become—improvement is inevitable at this point, and you can only add to your psychological framework of understanding, it will never go away. Once learnt, it can never be unlearnt. Good luck for your interview, and please remember that to be a good candidate, all you can be is your authentic self. That's all you need to be. Just you.

Index

Figures and boxes are indicated by an italic *f* and *b* following the page number.